Cardiorespiratory Fitness - New Topics

Edited by Hasan Sözen

Published in London, United Kingdom

Cardiorespiratory Fitness - New Topics
http://dx.doi.org/10.5772/intechopen.100928
Edited by Hasan Sözen

Contributors
Mirjam Močnik, Nataša Marčun Varda, Júlio Costa, Fábio Y. Nakamura, Jia-Ping Wu, Abirlal Sen, Riki Tesler, Dan Wang, Jun Ren, Kaiyuan Qu, Mingming Yang, Xin Yang, Anqi Lu, Paraschiva Postolache, Ştefan Săndulache, Constantin Ghimuş, Alexandru Nechifor, Adilson Marques, Miguel Peralta, Duarte Henriques-Neto, Sandra Martins, Jacquline C. Vadasseril, Theyamma Joseph, Hasan Sözen

First published in London, United Kingdom, 2023 by IntechOpen
IntechOpen is the global imprint of INTECHOPEN LIMITED, registered in England and Wales, registration number: 11086078, 5 Princes Gate Court, London, SW7 2QJ, United Kingdom

British Library Cataloguing-in-Publication Data
A catalogue record for this book is available from the British Library

Additional hard and PDF copies can be obtained from orders@intechopen.com

Cardiorespiratory Fitness - New Topics
Edited by Hasan Sözen
p. cm.
Print ISBN 978-1-80356-239-1
Online ISBN 978-1-80356-240-7
eBook (PDF) ISBN 978-1-80356-241-4

Meet the editor

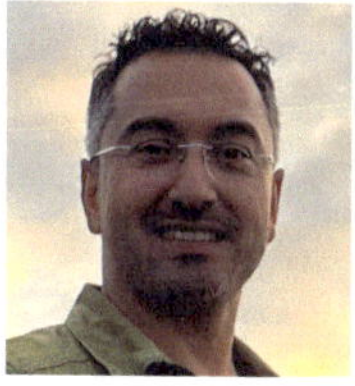

Dr. Hasan Sözen is an associate professor in the Sport Sciences Faculty, University of Ordu, Türkiye. His primary research interests include sport and exercise physiology, physical fitness, and athletes' health. Dr. Sözen received his Ph.D. from the Health Science Institute, Department of Physical Education and Sport, Ondokuz Mayıs University, Türkiye. He completed a post-doctoral fellowship at the Department of Biomedical Sciences for Health, University of Milan, Italy. The fellowship was supported by the Scientific and Technological Research Council of Türkiye.

Contents

Preface

Physical inactivity is considered the most important risk factor for cardiovascular diseases. Cardiorespiratory fitness (CRF), which refers to the ability of the circulatory and respiratory systems to provide oxygen during physical activity, is an important component of physical fitness and can be enhanced by regular physical activity. Lower CRF is associated with higher risks of Alzheimer's disease and cardiovascular diseases such as type 2 diabetes, hypertension, obesity, depression, poor physical fitness level, vascular dementia, and metabolic syndrome. In addition, CRF is inversely related to depression severity and cancer mortality.

This book includes nine chapters on CRF. Chapter 1 by Dr. Wang et al., "Cardiorespiratory Benefits of Exercise", examines the benefits of exercise on the cardiorespiratory system. Chapter 2 by Dr. Postolache et al., "Assessment of Exercise Capacity: A Key Element in Pulmonary Rehabilitation", discusses issues related to pulmonary rehabilitation, exercise capacity, and physical training in patients with CARF. Chapter 3 by Dr. Marques et al., "Promoting Cardiorespiratory Fitness in Young People: The Importance of the School Context", offers suggestions for increasing the CRF levels of school-aged children. The authors emphasize the importance of physical education lessons and physical education teachers in schools. Chapter 4 by Dr. Costa and Dr. Nakamura, "Assessment of Autonomic Cardiac Activity in Athletes", provides information about autonomic cardiac activity in athletes. It discusses the use of non-invasive and time-efficient methods to record and/or calculate heart rate variability in athletes. Chapter 5 by Dr. Wu, "Swimming Exercise-Induced Improvements in Cardiorespiratory Fitness (CRF) are Caused by Nitric Oxide Functional Adaptations in the Oxygen Transport System", argues that swimming exercise is a good way to increase metabolic rate and heat burning as well as improve heart rate and oxygen circulation. The chapter summarizes the roles of physiological nitric oxide in improvements in cardiorespiratory fitness. Chapter 6 by Dr. Močnik and Dr. Varda, "The Role of Cardiorespiratory Fitness in Children with Cardiovascular Risk", provides valuable and comprehensive information about the benefits of physical activity on children with cardiovascular risk to prevent further reduction of cardiorespiratory fitness and the development of other comorbidities. Chapter 7 by Dr. Sen and Dr. Baruah, "Effect of Hypertension on ECG Parameters," examines the relationship between ECG variables and blood pressure in medical school students. Chapter 8 by Dr. Joseph and Dr. Vadasseril, "Diabetes – A Silent Killer: A Threat for Cardiorespiratory Fitness", discusses type 2 diabetes mellitus, including its prevalence, risk factors, signs and symptoms, pathophysiology, and pathogenesis, as well as underlying mechanisms of diabetes as a disease, its acute and chronic complications, and measures to improve cardiorespiratory fitness and control diabetes. Finally, Chapter 9 by the editor, "Relationship Between Vastus Lateralis Electromyography Activation and VO_{2max} Values Obtained in Bicycle Ergometry", presents an experimental study investigating the relationship between the maximum oxygen consumption values obtained from a bicycle ergometer and the EMG activity values of the vastus lateralis muscle during the test.

On behalf of myself and all the contributing authors, I would like to thank Author Service Manager Mrs. Karla Skuliber at IntechOpen for her great support in preparing this book. I hope that readers will find *Cardiorespiratory Fitness – New Topics* to be a useful resource.

Hasan Sözen
Sport Sciences Faculty,
University of Ordu,
Ordu, Türkiye

Chapter 1

Cardiorespiratory Benefits of Exercise

Dan Wang, Kaiyuan Qu, Mingming Yang, Xin Yang, Anqi Lu and Jun Ren

Abstract

Abundant evidence proved that the amount of habitual exercise and the level of cardiorespiratory fitness (CRF) are inversely related to the risk of cardiovascular morbidity and mortality. In this chapter, you can learn about the cardiorespiratory benefits of exercise, involving: (1) delay the development of cardiovascular disease (CVD) affecting many of the standard cardiorespiratory diseases risk factors, such as plasma lipids, especially high-density lipoprotein cholesterol, fasting glucose levels, blood and hypertension control; (2) improve the cardiac output (CO) and the CRF of different ages. However, certain kind of exercise might not be applicable to cardiac patients, since high-intensity, high-volume exercise may increase all-cause mortality among these patients. At present, the American College of Sports Medicine (ACSM) recommends that aerobic exercise (AE) and resistance exercise (RE) two or three times a week is related to better physical function at different ages, improvement of muscle strength, body composition and, especially, CRF.

Keywords: fitness, cardiorespiratory, exercise, risk factor, insulin resistance, hypertension

1. Introduction

According to the statistics data, noncommunicable diseases (NCDs) such as cardiovascular disease (CVD), diabetes, and cancer are still on the rise [1, 2]. NCD resulted in more than 70% of all deaths globally, and there were about 41 million people killed in 2016 [3]. The majority of these deaths were due to CVD [3]. CVD accounts for 44% of these deaths, which translates to about 30% of all deaths [3]. CVD includes coronary artery disease, hypertensive heart disease, stroke, and thrombosis [4]. The risk factors for CVD are varied, such as high levels of plasma lipids and fasting glucose, lack of physical activity, and especially hypertension [4, 5].

Hypertension is one of the most fatal but preventable CVD worldwide [6]. The increased blood pressure is the main risk for death and disability which roughly accounts for 10% of medical healthcare expenditure [7, 8]. Around 40% of adults aged 25 years or older have hypertension, with an estimated 51% of stroke and 45% of heart disease caused by increased blood pressure [7, 9]. Hypertension may also contribute to complications in other prominent conditions such as coronary artery disease, thrombosis, and diabetes mellitus [10]. Moreover, the United Nations developed a target to decrease the incidence rate of nine chronic disease by 2025, of which four were related directly or indirectly to hypertension [9]. According to the statistics data, approximately 50% of hypertension was attributable to the lack of physical activity, 30% to high dietary salt, 15% to low dietary potassium, and 5% to excess alcohol intake [9]. For instance, physically inactive middle-aged women have been reported to have a 52% increase in all-cause mortality and a doubling in cardiovascular-related mortality [11]. In the general population, improving cardiorespiratory fitness (CRF) is a key countermeasure in the prevention of cardiorespiratory diseases and mortality [12, 13]. A study has shown that physical activity was associated with a risk reduction of more than 50% of CVD [14].

Due to the diversity of CVD, studies usually assess only some of the risk factors [15]. It is hard to issue specific recommendations for each CVD [15]. The American College of Sports Medicine (ACSM) suggested aerobic exercise (AE) of moderate intensity for five or more days per week with 30–60 min per session, or three or more vigorous-intensity exercise sessions with 20–60 min per session [16].

Whether physical activity had an effect on cardiovascular fitness and the magnitude of this effect would depend primarily on the frequency, intensity, type, and duration of the exercise [17, 18]. Physical activity can be classified in different ways, such as AE and resistance exercise (RE). AE is the type of exercise in which oxygen is utilized by working muscles [19]. It increases heart rate and energy consumption by dynamic repetitive contractions of major muscle groups [19]. AE is usually performed at a moderate intensity for 30–45 min in the form of continuous running, cycling, jogging, or swimming [20]. RE is the physical activity in which effort is spent against a specific resistive force and which is especially designed to increase muscle strength and endurance [21, 22]. AE has more benefits than RE on the increase of cardiovascular fitness [23]. For instance, AE usually affects all of the risk factors for CVD, including hypertension, plasma lipids, fasting glucose, and so on [24]. However, regular participation in RE can promote cardiovascular fitness by reducing body fat, increasing metabolic rate, lowering blood pressure and cholesterol levels, and increasing glucose tolerance [23, 24]. Moreover, RE can also improve CVD risk factors such as glucose metabolism and insulin sensitivity [24]. The higher muscle strength level is associated with better cardiometabolic, lower all-cause mortality, and fewer CVD events [1, 12]. Thus, AE and RE can be a good choice to promote cardiovascular fitness.

In conclusion, CVD remain the leading cause of death in the industrialized world. Fortunately, as an important part of health-related fitness, the level of cardiovascular fitness is inversely related to the risk of cardiovascular morbidity and mortality. Both AE and RE can increase cardiovascular fitness to a certain extent. Finally, before formulating an exercise plan, an appropriate health manager (such as a primary therapist, internist, or cardiologist) should be consulted to ensure the safety of exercise.

There were strong evidence supporting the cardiovascular health benefits associated with daily physical activity and exercise. Population-based studies have demonstrated that high levels of daily physical activity were associated with a lower risk of cardiovascular events and CVD mortality [25]. Exercise has positive physiologic effects on cardiovascular health, including but not limited to its impact on plasma lipids, especially high-density lipoprotein (HDL) cholesterol, insulin resistance, and hypertension control [26].

2. Risk factors for cardiovascular disease

2.1 High-density lipoprotein cholesterol

The primary driver of CVD development in humans appears to be the elevated level of blood cholesterol [27]. The same lipoprotein particles carry dietary and endogenous lipids. Chylomicrons transport dietary lipids, whereas low-density lipoproteins (LDLs) and high-density lipoproteins (HDLs) transport endogenous lipids. Triglycerides (also known as triglyceride-rich lipoproteins [TRLs]) made in the liver and intestines are transported to capillary beds by very low-density lipoproteins (VLDLs), where they serve as a source of energy for the target tissues [28]. The main method for moving cholesterol from a lesion site back to the liver is through HDL cholesterol. HDL reduces the development of plaque by a process known as "reverse cholesterol transfer" [29]. In addition, VLDL particles cannot pass through the endothelium wall due to their size, while LDL particles can pass through. However, in circulation, VLDLs have the potential to undergo hydrolysis along the luminal surface of capillaries, resulting in the production of free fatty acids and TRL remnants, which are higher in cholesterol than LDLs [29]. These leftovers are capable of being ingested by macrophages without being oxidized and are thus thought to exert a potent atherogenic effect [28]. Therefore, by modifying the lipid "profile," CVD risk can be decreased (i.e. lowering serum levels of LDL and triglycerides, and increasing HDL cholesterol).

Evidence from the last several decades supported the notion that exercise training has a favorable effect on the blood lipid profile [30]. One comprehensive review found that moderate to high intensity of AE increased the HDL cholesterol level (mean change across the studies reviewed was +4.6%) [31], in which diet was held constant for the participants. In a large randomized controlled trial, Kraus et al. [32] investigated the effects of AE of different volume and intensity on blood lipids. They randomly assigned 111 men and women with mild to moderate dyslipidemia into four groups: a high volume (jogging about 32 km/week) of high-intensity exercise (65–85% of peak oxygen consumption) and a low volume (jogging about 19.2 km/week) of high-intensity exercise (40–55% of peak oxygen consumption). In comparison with groups that engaged in low intensity/volumes of exercise, the high-intensity/high-volume exercise group showed a significant increase in the level of HDL cholesterol (+0.11378 mmol/l) and a decrease in triglycerides (−0.7344 mg/dl), but no significant change in the level of LDL cholesterol. Additionally, O'Donovan et al. [33] found that previously sedentary but healthy males who underwent 24 weeks of high-intensity (80% of aerobic capacity) AE had a significant decrease in LDL cholesterol levels, but not after low-intensity (60%) AE. A more recent metaanalysis [30] found that high-intensity aerobic interval training (i.e. periods of high-intensity exercise interspersed with periods of active/passive recovery) was more effective than moderate-intensity continuous exercise at raising HDL cholesterol levels in subclinical or clinical populations, independent of dietary or pharmaceutical interventions (e.g. healthy or obese individuals taking medications). Meanwhile, RE (i.e. strength exercises using body weight or external resistance) with greater volume of exercise (e.g. more sets and repetitions), but not necessarily greater intensity (e.g. higher loads), has been proven to significantly reduce the level of LDL cholesterol and triglycerides [24].

In addition, exercise enhances the skeletal muscle's capacity to utilize lipids as the main dietary source, which leads to a decrease in plasma lipid levels [34]. The upregulation of lipoprotein lipase, which hydrolyzes triglycerides into free fatty acids and encourages cellular uptake of TRL remnants, or lecithin cholesterol acyltransferase, which is involved in HDL cholesterol formation and, consequently, reverse cholesterol transport, may be used to partially achieve this goal. According to one previous research, an energy expenditure threshold (i.e. roughly 1000 kcal) must be met to elicit enhanced lipoprotein lipase activity in well-trained men [35]. This threshold may differ for different people based on their exercise history, disease condition (healthy vs. hypercholesterolemic), exercise intensity, age, sex, and type of exercise.

2.2 Insulin resistance

Insulin resistance is a significant predictor of CVD in patients with type 2 diabetes, since it is linked to the cluster of CVD risk factors mentioned earlier (high cholesterol and high blood pressure) [36]. The β cells of the pancreas secrete more insulin when an individual is insulin-resistant due to impaired glucose metabolism [37]. Vascular smooth muscle cells grow and proliferate when insulin levels are high [38]. This is due to the fact that elevated insulin level triggers the inflammatory pathways [39], which reduces nitric oxide levels and stimulates the secretion of endothelin-1; this in turn encourages vasoconstriction and atherogenesis [40]. Exercise might not be sufficient as a stand-alone treatment, as suboptimal diets are the primary lifestyle factors for insulin resistance. However, there were evidence showing significant beneficial impact of exercise on the insulin resistant state [41].

A series of research provided strong evidence for the efficacy of exercise in the treatment of type 2 diabetes. Boulé et al. [42] reviewed seven randomized controlled trials which compared the treatment effects of AE intervention (an average of 50 min per session and 3 sessions per week for 20 weeks) and control group (non-exercise) on patients with type 2 diabetes. As expected, the exercise intervention led to an approximate 12% increase in aerobic fitness compared with that in the controls. Exercise with higher intensity produced greater improvements in aerobic fitness and blood glucose control as defined by the reduction in glycated hemoglobin (HbA1c). However, exercise volume expressed as total weekly energy expenditure neither predicted the change in aerobic capacity nor in HbA1c. Later, this research group [43] further suggested that a threshold of 150 min of weekly structured exercise must be achieved for the significant reduction in HbA1c. An updated meta-analysis reported that patients with a higher level of HbA1c at the beginning of an intervention would experience a greater reduction in HbA1c, besides the magnitude of the reduction was associated with the volume of weekly AE or combined exercise (CE), but not the volume or intensity of RE [44]. However, Church et al. [45] demonstrated that patients with type 2 diabetes (HbA1c levels above 6.5%) involved in moderate-intensity AE (i.e. 150 min/week at 50–80% of the maximum intensity) combined with RE twice weekly for 9 months presented superior HbA1c decrement compared to those engaged in aerobic or resistance exercise alone.

Together, these data suggested that a minimum dose of approximately 150 min of accumulated exercise over the course of a week may be required to significantly influence the insulin resistant state. Additional beneficial effects may be achieved by increasing the intensity of AE. Resistance training (RT) may be most impactful when practiced in combination with an AE.

The mechanisms of exercise ameliorating diabetes have been well studied [46]. Exercise is emphasized as a therapeutic cornerstone for individuals with metabolic illnesses such as diabetes mellitus, as exercise-stimulated glucose absorption is preserved in insulin-resistant muscle [46]. Through the simultaneous enhancement of three crucial processes, including delivery, transport across the muscle membrane, and intracellular flow through metabolic pathways (glycolysis and glucose oxidation), exercise increases the absorption of glucose by up to 50 times [46]. Due to the complexity of the signaling pathways that regulate glucose uptake to ensure the maintenance of muscle energy supply during physical activity, the available data suggested that no single signal transduction pathway can fully account for the regulation of any of these important procedures [46]. Increased blood flow proportionate to exercise intensity caused an increase in glucose supply to working muscles, and an increase in skeletal muscle perfusion was related to the increase in glucose uptake [47]. Furthermore, it has been reported [48] that following just one cycling exercise session (i.e. 45–60 min at 60–70% of one's maximum effort), glucose transporter 4 (GLUT-4) concentrations were elevated by about 70% in comparison to baseline in both apparently healthy people and patients with type 2 diabetes. The glucose transporter known as GLUT-4 is responsible for facilitating the passage of plasma glucose into muscle and fat cells. Finally, it was discovered that GLUT-4 activity was closely related to the cell metabolism of glucose. During exercise, glycogen is the primary energy source. In order to produce the adenosine triphosphate required for exercise, glycogen is gradually hydrolyzed to blood glucose as activity continues and glycogen stores become exhausted [46]. In conclusion, exercise is an efficient treatment for CVD by simultaneously boosting the elements that enhance glucose delivery, transport, and metabolism.

2.3 Hypertension

Hypertension is one of the most fatal but preventable CVD worldwide [49]. It tends to coexist with hypercholesterolemia [50]. Hypertension is closely associated with inactive lifestyle. Exercise was shown to delay the development of hypertension. AE was recommended by the American Heart Association/American College of Cardiology [51], the European Society of Hypertension/European Society of Cardiology [52], and the Canadian Hypertension Education Program [53] as the first-line treatment for the prevention, treatment, and control of elevated blood pressure or hypertension. Numerous randomized controlled trials supported an average drop in blood pressure of 5–7 mm Hg following AE programs [54]. These governing bodies all agreed that exercise should be undertaken on the majority of days of the week, if not every day. It was founded on the discovery of post-exercise hypotension, or the sudden drop in blood pressure that occurs after a single, severe episode of AE [55]. This drop in blood pressure can sustain for a full day [56]. The drop of the resting blood pressure following long-term AE training was correlated with the drop of the blood pressure after acute exercise [57]. Furthermore, the magnitude of drop of the blood pressure appears to be dose-dependent, which was supported by Eicher et al. who measured ambulatory blood pressure in 45 pre- or stage 1 hypertensive men after they completed low-intensity (40% of peak oxygen consumption), moderate-intensity (60% of peak oxygen consumption), and high-intensity (100% of peak oxygen consumption) exercise, respectively [58]. High-intensity exercise resulted in a blood pressure drop of 11.7/4.9 mm Hg, followed by moderate-intensity exercise (5.4/2.0 mm Hg), and low-intensity exercise (2.8/1.5 mm Hg). A group of persons with resistant hypertension (e.g. blood pressure > 140/90 mm Hg despite using three antihypertensive medicines) who exercised at a moderate intensity three times per week for 8–12 weeks showed a significant decrease in ambulatory blood pressure

(6/3 mm Hg) [59]. Even middle-aged hypertension individuals who were deprived of antihypertensive medications experienced a significant drop in resting blood pressure (−16/−12 mm Hg) after moderate-intensity RT.

In conclusion, suggestions in practice for hypertension were as follows: (1) a dose-response relationship exists between AE intensity and blood pressure; (2) moderate-intensity exercise can be used to achieve clinically significant reduction in blood pressure among individuals with established hypertension but resistant to drug therapy; (3) reductions in blood pressure are observed across different exercise modalities [56].

The principal mechanism of exercise maintaining or lowering blood pressure was believed to be the reduction in total peripheral resistance. Exerciseinduced vascular and autonomic adaptations have been proposed to potentially provide major contributions to blood pressure control [60]. First, hypertensive patients show enhanced sympathetic control, which causes vasoconstriction of arterial beds and thus raises total peripheral resistance [61]. This could be induced by the heightened sensitivity of baroreceptor, which are located in the carotid sinus and aortic arch and are in charge of detecting changes in blood pressure [57]. Baroreceptor's sensitivity is influenced by exercise [62]. For instance, after 4 months of cycling exercise (three times per week at 70% of maximum capacity), the improvements in baroreflex control was corresponded to the reduction in blood pressure and muscle sympathetic nerve activity in a group of hypertensive patients, and their sensitivity was reset to those observed in normotensives [63]. Second, through the local vascular control mechanisms, exercise improves vascular function [64]. In particular, exercise reduces the bioavailability of endothelin-1, a vasoconstrictor, and increases the bioavailability of nitric oxide, a powerful vasodilator [65]. The endothelial cells secrete both of these two chemicals. Endothelial function improved as a result of exercise training, which improved the nitric oxide vasodilator [66]. A recent study [67] observed similar improvements in endothelial function among patients with prehypertension or hypertension who engaged in 8 weeks of aerobic, resistance, or combined exercise. Endothelin-1 concentrations were observed to be higher in older, normotensive women who had previously been sedentary (aged 61–69) than in younger women (aged 21–28) [68]. However, after 3 months of cycling activity (5 days per week), the concentrations were markedly lowered along with the blood pressure. Third, physical activity increases the compliance of large elastic arteries, the aorta, and carotids for instance, which attenuates the fluctuations of the pressure for each heartbeat. Left ventricular hypertrophy would arise from an increase in ventricular afterload caused by a decrease in arterial compliance. Following 3 months of AE training (4–6 days per week, at 70–75% of maximum capacity), an improvement in arterial compliance of the carotid artery was also noticed in middle to old age sedentary normotensive men (50 1 years) [69]. In contrast, people with isolated systolic hypertension did not experience any changes in systemic arterial compliance following 8 weeks (3 days per week) of moderate-intensity (65% of maximal capacity) cycling [70]. The carotid artery stiffness in a group of elderly hypertensives (68.2 ± 5.4 years) was unaffected by 20 weeks (3 days per week) of moderate-intensity (70% of the maximum capacity) AE [71]. Stewart et al. [72] found that while diastolic blood pressure improved following 6 months of combined aerobic and RE in a group of old (55–75 years) hypertensive patients, no changes in systolic blood pressure or aortic stiffness were observed. These findings may be related to genetic, dietary, or long-term training habits and did not provide insight into the effects of training in previously sedentary patients with isolated systolic hypertension. These conflicting data suggested that, in the future, we need to further investigate the effect of exercise on elastic vascular adherence.

3. Benefits of exercise on cardiovascular disease

3.1 Cardiac output

3.1.1 Four determinants of cardiac output

Cardiac output (CO) is the amount of blood pumped out of the left or right ventricle per minute, namely the product of heart rate and output of each stroke. It is expressed with liter/minute. If the heart rate was 75 times per minute, the CO would be 5–6 L in men and slightly lower in women. CO varies with people's metabolism rate and activity level. It increases with muscle movement, emotional agitation, pregnancy, etc., and is determined by the heart rate, myocardial contractility, preload, and afterload (**Figure 1**).

3.1.2 Heart rate

Heart rate refers to the frequency of heart contraction beats, or the number of beats per minute (bpm). When a person is at rest, heart rate is 60–100 times per minute (60–100 bpm). Heart rate will increase during exercise, and athletes with better cardiopulmonary function will have a slower heart rate than people without exercise experience. The age-predicted HRmax eq. (220-age) is commonly used as a basis for prescribing exercise programs. It is considered as a standard for achieving maximal exertion and as a clinical guide during diagnostic exercise testing. A direct percentage of HRmax or a fixed percentage of heart rate reserve (HRmax – heart rate at rest) is used as a basis for prescribing exercise intensity in both rehabilitation and disease prevention programs [73].

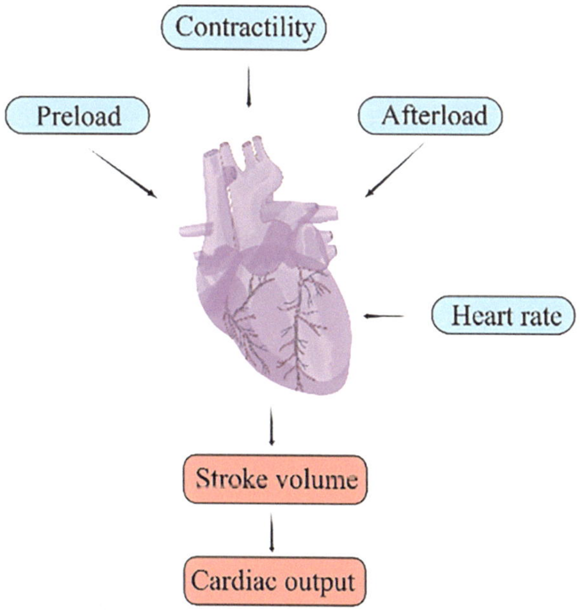

Figure 1.
Cardiac output. By Figdraw (www.figdraw.com).

Heart rate in adults depends on the activity of the sinoatrial node cells and constantly varies under the influence of a number of nonmodifiable and modifiable factors. The sinoatrial node cells are innervated by the parasympathetic fibers of the vagus and sympathetic nervous thoracic efferents and regulate the heart rate [74]. It was reported that increased all-cause mortality and cardiovascular risk events are associated with high heart rate, more so in men than in women. An increase of 10 beats per minute in a person's heart rate is associated with a 20% increase in cardiac death [75]. Heart rate recorded in elderly men has a strong predictive value in the survival to a very old age.

3.1.3 Contractility

Contractility is the inherent strength and vigor of the heart's contraction during systole. According to Starling's law, the heart will eject a greater stroke volume at greater filling pressures. Heart contraction is initiated by the action potential propagated from sinoatrial node cells [76]. Following which, Ca^{2+} influx through mainly L-type Ca^{2+} channels in the surface membrane promotes further release of stored Ca^{2+} from the sarcoplasmic reticulum (SR) via the SR Ca^{2+} release channel (the ryanodine receptor, RyR) by a process known as Ca^{2+}-induced Ca release. The two Ca^{2+} fluxes mentioned earlier combine to initiate contraction [77].

3.1.4 Preload

Preload is the filling pressure of the heart at the end of diastole. The greater the preload, the greater volume of blood will be in the heart at the end of diastole. Preload builds up during diastolic filling and stretches cardiomyocytes. Left atrial pressure (LAP) determines the volume of the heart at the end of diastole, which relates to the filling pressure (preload). The relationship of stroke volume index to LAP is usually plotted as Starling's law. Contractility and afterload modify this relationship.

3.1.5 Afterload

Afterload is the force against which the myocardial fibers must contact during the ejection phase of systole [78]. In response to a decrease in CO, the body's homeostatic system will attempt to maintain blood pressure by increasing vascular resistance in the system. When the preload reserve is reduced and the ventricles are hypocontractible, a decrease in afterload generally results in an increase in output [79]. By increasing output, hypotension will be countered, resulting in good clinical results.

3.2 Cardiorespiratory fitness

CRF refers to the capacity of the circulatory and respiratory systems to supply oxygen to skeletal muscle mitochondria for energy production needed during physical activity [80]. It is an intermediate variable between physical activity behavior and health outcomes and reflects the ability of many body organs (such as heart, lungs, and muscles) to generate energy during physical activity and exercise [81]. Maximal oxygen uptake (VO_{2max}) is considered the gold standard for CRF and can be estimated using either a maximal graded cardiopulmonary test or an indirect calculating method [82]. CRF is associated with CVD and is a strong independent predictor of all-cause mortality in adults [80]. Higher levels of CRF were associated with lower cardiovascular morbidity and all-cause mortality [83].

3.2.1 Physical activity and cardiorespiratory fitness

Physical activity and CRF were associated with health and quality of life, and even small improvements in physical fitness were associated with reduced CVD and all-cause mortality [84]. Based on the importance of physical activity to CRF, the current physical activity guidelines recommend that all adults engage in at least 150 min of moderate-intensity exercise or 75 min of vigorous-intensity exercise per week [84]. To improve CRF, current evidence suggests that physical exercise must achieve a minimum intensity of at least 45% of the oxygen absorption reserve in the general population and at least 70–80% in athletes [83]. Vigorous exercise was associated with greater improvements in VO_{2max} than moderate-intensity exercise [84].

3.2.2 Training type and cardiopulmonary fitness

In recent years, many studies have identified moderate-intensity continuous training (MICT), high-intensity interval training (HIIT), and high-intensity functional training (HIFT) as interventions for CRF [85, 86]. MICT is a traditional way to increase physical activity, and its effectiveness depends on training for longer periods of time [86]. HIIT is defined as intervals of alternating high-intensity and low-intensity activity, or short bursts of passive recovery [82]. HIIT is recommended because of its short duration (20–30 min) and high efficiency in improving physical fitness and health parameters [86]. HIFT is an exercise modality that emphasizes functional, multi-joint movements that can be tuned to any fitness level and stimulate muscle replenishment more than traditional exercise. As a relatively new training form, HIFT is often compared to HIIT, yet the two are distinct [85].

3.2.3 Cardiac output and cardiopulmonary fitness

Research evidence suggested that higher CRF is associated with higher CO through augmented stroke volume or heart rate, and lower systolic blood pressure, pulmonary arterial pressure, and vascular resistance [87]. In cardiopulmonary exercise testing (CPET), peak oxygen uptake (VO_2peak) is the gold standard for CRF measurement, and research evidence showed that the decline of VO_2peak is mainly related to a lower maximum CO [87].

3.3 Improve the cardiac output and the cardiorespiratory fitness

3.3.1 Preschool children (ages 3–5 years)

Regular physical activity in preschoolers is essential for normal growth and development, providing immediate and long-term benefits for physical and mental health, while the World Health Organization recommends that typically developing children between the ages of 3 and 5 years should be physically active for 3 h a day [88].

An important point of enhancing cardiopulmonary fitness is to execute moderate-to high-intensity physical activity (MVPA) [89], and aerobic training has been proved to effectively improve the VO_{2max} of preschool children [90]. According to a study of meta-analysis, preschool children are mainly focused on improving coordination and perception, such as 40 min of moderate-to-higher intensity physical activity (brisk walking, jogging, jumping, squatting, crawling, and other alternative exercises) [91].

In conclusion, moderate- to high-intensity physical activity and aerobic training can improve the CRF of preschool children.

3.3.2 Children and adolescents (ages 6-17 years)

Enhancement of CRF has been identified as a key goal for reducing cardiovascular metabolic risk in children and adolescents [92]. A scientific statement from the American Heart Association indicates that high-intensity exercise, including high-intensity interval training, can improve cardiopulmonary fitness in adolescents [80]. At the same time, a study showed that HIIT is a better training methodology to improve CRF among healthy children and adolescents compared to MICT based on the characteristics and efficiency [82]. Secondly, a systematic review study found that HIIT influenced neuromuscular and an AE performance in children and adolescents, including jumping performance and the number of sit-ups [93]. Therefore, more and more research evidence suggested that HIIT may improve the cardiopulmonary fitness of children and adolescents.

3.3.3 Young adults (ages 18-44 years)

As an indicator of CRF, high VO_{2max} indicated a relatively great level of aerobic capacity which was associated with better physical performance [94]. In the general adult population, HIIT is highly effective as an intervention to enhance CRF, but not significantly for the adult population with exercise habits [94]. There are also studies on RT as an intervention program to enhance CRF. However, the effect of cardiovascular adaptation from RT was controversial, and some researches believed that RT had no benefits on the increase of CRF [95]. A study suggested that RT could not promote CRF mainly because of insufficient training intensity [96]. However, Keith believed that in the long run, high-intensity RT produces more physiological adaptations and contributes to observed improvements in cardiovascular health, such as increased mitochondrial enzymes, mitochondrial proliferation, and conversion of type ii X muscle fibers to Type ii A muscle fibers, and vascular remodeling [97]. Therefore, high-intensity RT can improve CRF. Currently, endurance exercise is well recognized to improve CRF and cardiometabolic risk factors.

In the general adult population, HIIT, high-intensity RT, and endurance exercise can improve CRF.

3.3.4 Middle-aged (ages 45-59 years) adults

HIIT has been promoted as a superior, time-saving exercise strategy to enhance CRF in the middle-aged [98]. A systematic review of evidence suggested that both interval training and MICT could significantly improve CRF in middle-aged and elderly people; however, MICT has no significant effect on improving VO_{2max} in middle-aged compared with HIIT and sprint interval training. This may be due to their exercise intensity and a substantially reduced training volume and lower time commitment [99]. Therefore, compared with MICT, HIIT is better for promoting maximal oxygen uptake in middle-aged adults. Circular resistance training also showed significant effects on improving circular resistance training, strength, and optimizing body composition in middle-aged [100]. In the middle-aged adults, HIIT,

MICT, and circular resistance training can all produce adaptability, so the above training methods can be considered for exercise programs involving the middle-aged [101]. However, HIIT is still the preferred training method.

3.3.5 Younger-old (60-70) adults

With the increase of age, it was documented that the cognitive function of the elderly group declined. Besides, attention control was also affected (such as talking, listening, and writing while driving), which led to the decline of executive function (such as driving and walking) [102]. In fact, higher CRF has been shown to be related to brain structural modification, changes in functional connectivity and higher cerebral blood volume that could enhance cognitive function [102]. Physical training, especially AE (40 min or so) for 8–72 weeks, has been shown to be effective in improving cognitive function and regulating CRF in older adults [103]. Secondly, a systematic review suggested that HIIT and MICT can improve the CRF in younger-old adults, but HIIT is more effective at improving brachial artery vascular function than MICT, perhaps due to its tendency to positively influence CRF [104]. In RT, multi-articular RT has a better effect on CRP than single-articular RT [97]. These positive effects may be due to training intensity because high-intensity RT increases basal metabolic rate and fat oxidation. The multi-articular RT belongs to high intensity [97].

In conclusion, physical exercise, HIIT, and multi-articular RT are more likely to enhance CRF in younger-old adults.

3.3.6 Older-old (70+) adults

Aging is associated with a decline in CRF and VO_{2max} (maximum oxygen intake per unit of time). In healthy older adults over 70 years, aging accelerates the decline in VO_2peak values (the highest point in oxygen uptake) by an average of 20–25% per decade. Furthermore, cognition, physical abilities (such as muscle strength, balance, and cardiovascular endurance), body function, and independence generally decline with aging [105]. At the same time, increased age is associated with increased risk of injuries during daily living activities and CVD [106].

Recent studies with small sample size and less intervention time showed that HIIT not only increased CRF in healthy elderly people but also had a positive effect on muscle strength, oxidative stress, inflammation, and insulin sensitivity [107]. RT has not been considered as a training method to improve CRF, but some studies have found that RT may be viable means to improve cardiopulmonary endurance in the elderly [108]. This may be due to increased oxidative enzyme activities or by increasing leg strength so that muscle weakness does not preclude achievement of VO_2peak [108]. MICT and RT were superior to HIIT in enhancing executive cognitive function in the elderly, while HIIT was more conducive to improving physical endurance [109].

In conclusion, HIIT is still an optimal training method to improve CRF in the elderly, while aerobic training, MICT, and RT can also include in the intervention program.

As outlined above, AE, RE, and CE were suggested as the effective exercise intervention for people with CVD risk. Detailed information related to the exercise prescription would be discussed in this section. Exercise prescription includes six components: frequency, intensity, time, type, volume, and progression (FITT-VP). Frequency describes how often one executes exercise, intensity signifies how hard the exercise is, time refers to the total time spent on exercise (length of each training session, daily or weekly exercise), type stands for what kind of exercise one chooses to participate, volume is determined by a combination of frequency, intensity, and time, and progression means the adjustment of the frequency, intensity, and time of the exercise to gradually achieve the exercise goal [20, 110].

4. Exercise prescription for the improvement of cardiovascular fitness

4.1 Aerobic exercise

In AE, the large muscles move in a rhythmic manner for a sustained period. AE causes the heart rate to increase and breathing to become more labored [19]. AE is usually performed in a moderate intensity for 30–45 min in the form of continuous running, cycling, jogging, or swimming [20].

4.1.1 Frequency of aerobic exercise

To promote or maintain health/fitness, preschool-aged children should be physically active throughout the day to enhance growth and development [111]. Children and adolescents aged 6 through 17 years should include physical activity at least 3 days a week [111]. The ACSM recommended moderate-intensity AE for most adults at least 5 days per week, or at least 3 days of vigorous AE per week, or a combination of moderate and vigorous exercise 3–5 days a week [110]. Some adults can improve their health with moderate to vigorous activity only 1–2 days a week [110]. However, irregular vigorous exercise may increase the risk of cardiovascular events, and therefore 1–2 days of exercise a week was not recommended for most adults [20]. This recommendation for most adults also applies to older adults. It is important to note that older people should determine their level of effort in physical activity according to their physical condition [20].

4.1.2 The intensity of aerobic exercise

The intensity of AE can be divided into absolute intensity and relative intensity. Absolute intensity refers to the amount of energy consumed during the activity, regardless of people's CRF or aerobic ability [110]. It is expressed in the metabolic equivalent (MET) of task units; 1 MET is equivalent to resting metabolic rate or energy consumption during wakefulness and meditation [20]. Relative intensity refers to the degree of effort required to carry out an activity relative to a person's ability [20]. Since the measurement of absolute intensity does not take individual factors into account, such as weight, gender, and fitness level, it may lead to misclassification of exercise intensity [112]. Therefore, relative intensity is more appropriate in the evaluation of exercise intensity, especially for the elderly [20]. There are several commonly used methods for estimating relative exercise intensity during AE: oxygen uptake reserve (VO_2R), heart rate reserve (HRR), percent of the maximum HR (%HRmax), $\%VO_{2max}$, and MET [113]. **Table 1** shows the approximate classification of AE intensity commonly used in practice.

In cardiovascular regulation and disease prevention, low-, moderate-, and vigorous-intensity exercise have all exhibited some degrees of health benefit [114].

Aerobic exercise				
Relative intensity				**Absolute intensity**
Intensity	%HRR or %VO_2R	%HR_{max}	%VO_{2max}	METs
Very light	<30	<57	<37	<2
Light	30–39	57–63	37-45	2.0–2.9
Moderate	40–59	64–76	46-63	3.0–5.9
Vigorous	60–89	77–95	64-90	6.0–8.7
Near-maximal to maximal	≥90	≥96	≥91	≥8.8

The table was adapted from the American College of Sports Medicine [112]. HRmax: maximal heart rate; HRR: heart rate reserve; MET: metabolic equivalent; VO_{2max}: maximal volume of oxygen consumed per minute; VO_2R: oxygen uptake reserve.

Table 1.
Classification of exercise intensity: relative and absolute intensity for aerobic exercise.

A significant dose-response relationship exists between exercise intensity and overall cardiovascular benefit [115]. Compared with moderate intensity, vigorous-intensity exercise takes less time to obtain the same benefits of improving CRF and preventing CVD. For example, exercise at moderate intensity for 30 min produces roughly the same as that of 15 min of vigorous-intensity exercise [20]. The study found that exercise performed at higher relative intensity led to a greater increase in aerobic capacity and greater cardiac protection than exercise at moderate intensity [116]. However, vigorous activity can also acutely and transiently increase the risk of sudden cardiac death and myocardial infarction in susceptible people [117]. Consequently, it was recommended that people of different ages should engage in moderate (40–59% HRR or VO_2R) to vigorous (60–89% HRR or VO_2R) AE; people in poor health should undergo low- (30–39% HRR or VO_2R) to moderate-intensity AE to improve CRF and prevent CVD [20]. It is noted that children, the elderly, and the frail should exercise under the guidance of caregivers, doctors, and professional trainers to ensure safety [118].

4.1.3 Time of aerobic exercise

Children younger than 6 years undergo periods of rapid growth and development. The recommended duration of exercise for preschool-aged children is 3 h per day of activity of all intensities [111]. School-aged children and adolescents are in the critical periods for developing movement skills, learning healthy habits, and establishing a firm foundation for lifelong health [20]. Aerobic physical activity for 60 min or more per day at moderate or vigorous intensity was recommended for the majority of them [20]. Most adults are recommended to exercise at least 30–60 min at moderate intensity per day (>150 min per week), or at least 20–60 min at vigorous intensity per day (>75 min per week), or execute a combination of moderate- and vigorous-intensity exercise [110]. Older adults should achieve 150 min of moderate-intensity AE per week [112]. The recommended amount of exercise can be completed by continuous or cumulative time over the course of a day with multiple activities, but at least 10 min each time [119]. Even if the duration of exercise is below the minimum recommended amount, there may be benefits for some people, especially for sedentary people [118].

Exercise type	Recommended population	Example
Aerobic exercise requiring minimal skill or physical fitness	Most people	Walking, jogging, recreational biking, water aerobics, slow dancing, and skip rope
High-intensity aerobic exercise requiring a minimum of skill	People who exercise regularly and/ or at least moderately fit	Jogging, running, rowing, water aerobics, spinning, elliptical, stair climbing, and speed dancing
Aerobic exercise that requires skill	Skilled people and/or at least moderately fit	Swimming, cross-country skiing, and ice skating
Leisure sports	People with regular exercise and/ or at least moderate fitness level	Tennis, badminton, basketball, soccer, downhill skiing, and hiking

Table 2.
Aerobic exercise to improve cardiorespiratory fitness [112, 115].

4.1.4 Type of aerobic exercise

Periodic, large-muscle-involved, low-skill-required, at least moderate-intensity of AE was recommended for most people to promote health and CRF [110]. Sports that require other skills and a higher level of fitness are only recommended for those with appropriate skills and fitness [112]. **Table 2** categorizes AE according to different intensity and skills required.

4.1.5 Volume of aerobic exercise

Findings from epidemiological and randomized clinical trials showed that health/ fitness benefits increase with physical activity [110]. Although it was not clear whether there was a maximum or minimum volume of exercise to obtain health/fitness benefits, a total energy expenditure of not less than 500–1000 METs-min/week was strongly associated with lower CVD morbidity and mortality [110]. Therefore, a reasonable volume of exercise recommended for most people is ≥500–1000 METs-min/week. This volume of exercise was equivalent to approximately 150 min/week of moderate intensity exercise or physical activity per week [110]. It was noted that smaller volume of exercise (e.g. 4 kcal/kg or 330 kcal/week) may also provide health/ fitness benefits for some individuals, especially those with low fitness. Therefore, it was not possible to establish a recommendation of minimum volume of exercise [20].

4.1.6 Progression of aerobic exercise

The progression of the AE program depends on the frequency, intensity, and time (FIT) of the exercise [110]. When implementing program progression, this can be accomplished by the increase of either one or the free combination of the FIT principles of exercise prescription that the exerciser can tolerate [110]. At the beginning of the exercise program, it is recommended to gradually increase the time/duration of exercise (e.g. the duration of each training session) [110]. A more reasonable progression recommended for the general adult population is to extend the time of each training session by 5–10 min every 1–2 week for the first 4–6 week of the program. After regular exercise at least 1 month for older adults and those with lower fitness, the FIT can be gradually increased over the next 4–8 months until achieving the recommended frequency and intensity [20]. The exerciser's response should be observed after any adjustment to the exercise prescription for adverse reactions, such as shortness of breath, fatigue, and muscle soreness after exercise, and the exercise volume should be reduced when the exerciser was unable to tolerate the adjusted program [120].

4.2 Resistance exercise

RE refers to the active exercise of muscles when overcoming external resistance [121]. RE makes the muscles of the body work or withstand the force or weight exerted, thus improving muscle strength and endurance [20]. RE usually used self-weights, extra weights, air resistance equipment, and elastic bands or dumbbells for resistance to strengthen muscle groups in various parts of the body [20]. Regular participation in RE promotes cardiopulmonary fitness by reducing body fat, increasing metabolic rate, and lowering blood pressure and cholesterol levels [24]. RE improves CVD risk factors such as glucose metabolism and insulin sensitivity [122]. Thus, higher muscle strength level is associated with better cardiometabolic, lower all-cause mortality, and fewer CVD events [123].

4.2.1 Frequency of resistance exercise

Optimal RE frequency depends on several factors such as volume, intensity, and type of exercise, level of conditioning, fatigue recovery ability, and number of muscle groups trained per workout session [124]. According to previous research, RE is appropriate for most people for 2–3 days per week for the major muscle groups (e.g. upper limb, lower limb, chest, back, and core) in the body [125]. Following a period of RE, progression to intermediate level of training is recommended. This could be exercise at a frequency of 3–4 days per week (if trained for the whole body, 3 days a week was required; if trained in a split way, 4 days a week was required) [126]. A rest period of 48–72 h between sessions is needed to optimally promote the cellular/molecular adaptations that stimulate muscle hypertrophy and are associated gains in strength [127].

4.2.2 The intensity of resistance exercise

The recommendation for intensity of RE was as follows: (1) preschool-aged children use body weight exercises to ensure safety and allow for technical development; (2) <60% of 1 repetition maximum (RM) for children and adolescents; (3) 60–70% of 1 RM interval training for beginners; (4) 80% of 1 RM for experienced strength trainers; (5) 40–50% of 1 RM for older, very deconditioned, or frail individuals; (6) 40–50% of 1 RM for sedentary people [121].

4.2.3 Type of resistance exercise

Research has proven that different training type can be effective in RE for children and adolescents, including the use of one's own weight as resistance, the use of elastic bands, medicine balls, free weight equipment, and child-sized training equipment [128]. For most adults, many RE tools can be used to effectively improve muscle fitness, including free load, ropes, air resistance equipment, and elastic bands [121]. Older adults can use different types of fitness equipment, including weight training equipment, free weights (barbells and dumbbells), or household items such as plastic bottles filled with water [119]. RE should include multi-joint or compound exercises, which can mobilize multiple muscle groups to participate in sports (such as horizontal push, shoulder push, pull-down, arm flexion and extension, prone push-up, sit-up/ knee flexion, kick, and squat) [129]. Moreover, it should also include single-joint exercises, such as biceps curls, triceps extensions, quadriceps extensions, calf bending, heel lift, and core muscle group exercises (such as plate support and bridge) [124]. However, in order to maximize the training effect, we should focus on multi-joint exercise. Multi-joint movement is more complex, allowing more muscles to be involved in it and lift a heavier load [130]. It is recommended to separate the whole-body training and upper and lower limbs training. Separate training of muscle groups includes training of large muscle groups before small muscle groups, multi-joint training before single joints, and high-intensity training before low-intensity training [131]. In addition, pay attention to proper breathing during strength training, usually exhaling when lifting the weight and inhaling when putting it down [127].

4.2.4 Volume of resistance exercise

The volume of training can be accomplished by varying the number of practices per class, the number of repetitions per set, or the number of practices per set [121]. Research has shown that preschool-aged children and adolescents mostly use 1–3 sets of 6–12 repetitions for exercises [111]. For beginners and most adults, RT with 2–4 sets of 8–12 repetitions would be sufficient [20]. For older adults, RT with 1–3 sets of 8–12 repetitions in the beginning could effectively improve strength [132]. For RE of all ages, rest intervals of 2–3 min are most effective for achieving the desired increases in muscle strength and hypertrophy [110].

4.2.5 Progression of resistance exercise

After adapted the muscles to the original load through a RE program, muscle strength and volume can be continued to increase through overload or greater stimulation [127]. Exercisers can gradually increase the resistance, the number of repetitions, and frequency to reach the progression [127]. In general, increase the load by 2–10% (low percentage for small muscle mass exercises and high percentage for large muscle mass exercises) when the individual can complete the required workload once or twice in two consecutive sessions [110]. Note that when children and adolescents perform RE, the focus should be on the proper exercise technique, but not on how much weight to lift [20]. The elderly and frail should receive a health check from a doctor or provider before participating in RE. If necessary, seek supervision and guidance from a qualified fitness instructor to ensure exercise safety [110].

4.3 Combined exercise

The combination of aerobic and resistance exercise has been shown to have an additive effect on the enhancement of CRF and the reduction of the risk of CVD, allowing individuals to achieve greater and more comprehensive CVD health benefits [133]. Studies recommended at least two or more CE sessions per week for children and adolescents [134]. For most adults, CE is better performed at least 2–3 times per week for 30–60 min (15 or 30 min for AE and RE, respectively). AE can be conducted at 50–80% HRR for exercises such as cycling, elliptical, and treadmill. RE should be performed at 50–80% 1RM for two sets of 8–12 repetitions. The movements include muscle groups of the whole body, for example, leg press, hamstring curl, quadriceps extension, chest press, abdominal crunch, lower back extension, and torso rotation [135]. The FITT-VP of CE can refer to the aforementioned information.

5. Conclusion

CVD remains the leading cause of death in the industrialized world. Luckily, increased level of exercise and improved aerobic fitness can dramatically reduce CVD risk. Evidence from randomized controlled trials studies suggested that structured exercise confers cardio protection, delays the development of CVD, and influences many CVD risk factors, such as plasma lipids, especially high-density lipoprotein cholesterol, fasting glucose levels, and hypertension. A general understanding of these benefits can be supportive for physical activity and exercise promotion in health care settings.

CRF is an important part of health-related fitness. AE, RE, and CE can all improve CRF to a certain extent. Moreover, there are a wide range of forms of AE, RE, and CE, which can meet the needs of different groups for CRF enhancement and CVD prevention. Exercisers can choose the appropriate exercise for themselves based on the FITT-VP recommendations provided earlier. When exercising, start with a reasonable amount of exercise and make the process gradually. The elderly and the infirm should exercise under the guidance of doctors and professional coaches to ensure safety.

Fund

The research is funded by the program for Overseas High-level Talents at Shanghai Institutions of Higher Learning under Grant No. TP2019072, Natural Science Foundation of the Higher Education Institutions of Jiangsu Province under Grant No. 17KJB320008, Shanghai Key Lab of Human Performance (Shanghai University of Sport) under Grant No. 11DZ2261100, and Key project of "Science and Technology Winter Olympics" in national key research and development program (2021YFF0307105).

Author details

Dan Wang[1*], Kaiyuan Qu[1], Mingming Yangm[1], Xin Yang[1], Anqi Lu[1] and Jun Ren[2]

1 School of Elite Sport, Shanghai University of Sport, Shanghai, China

2 Shanghai Institute of Cardiovascular Diseases, Department of Cardiology, Zhongshan Hospital, Fudan University, Shanghai, China

*Address all correspondence to: wangdan@sus.edu.cn

References

[1] Alwan A, Maclean DR, Riley LM, et al. Monitoring and surveillance of chronic non-communicable diseases: Progress and capacity in high-burden countries. The Lancet. 2010;**376**:1861-1868. DOI: 10.1016/S0140-6736(10)61853-3

[2] Wagner KH, Brath H. A global view on the development of non communicable diseases. Preventive Medicine. 2012;**54**:38-41. DOI: 10.1016/j.ypmed.2011.11.012

[3] Verbrugghe J, Agten A, Eijnde BO, et al. Feasibility of high intensity training in nonspecific chronic low back pain: A clinical trial. Journal of Back & Musculoskeletal Rehabilitation. 2018;**31**:1-10. DOI: 10.3233/BMR-170810

[4] Yusuf, Reddy, Ounpuu, et al. Global burden of cardiovascular diseases: Part I: General considerations, the epidemiologic transition, risk factors, and impact of urbanization. Circulation 2001; 104:2746-2753. DOI: 10.1161/hc4601.099487

[5] Anderson KM, Odell PM, Wilson P, et al. Cardiovascular disease risk profiles. American Heart Journal. 1991;**121**:293-298. DOI: 10.1016/0002-8703(91)90861-B

[6] Williams B, Mancia G, Spiering W, et al. 2018ESC/ESH guidelines for the management of arterial hypertension. Journal of Hypertension. 2018;**36**:2284-2309. DOI: 10.1093/eurheartj/ehy339

[7] Lim, Stephen S, Theo, et al. A comparative risk assessment of burden of disease and injury attributable to 67 risk factors and risk factor clusters in 21 regions, 1990-2010: A systematic analysis for the Global Burden of Disease Study 2010. The Lancet. 2013;**380**:2224-2260. DOI: 10.1016/S0140-6736(12)61766-8

[8] Gaziano TA, Bitton A, Anand S, et al. The global cost of nonoptimal blood pressure. Journal of Hypertension. 2009;**27**:1472-1477. DOI: 10.1097/HJH.0b013e32832a9ba3

[9] Campbell, Norm RC, Niebylski, et al. Prevention and control of hypertension: Developing a global agenda. Current Opinion in Cardiology. 2014;**29**:324-330. DOI: 10.1097/HCO.0000000000000067

[10] Chen G, Mcalister FA, Walker RL, et al. Cardiovascular outcomes in Framingham participants with diabetes: The importance of blood pressure. Hypertension. 2011;**57**:891-897. DOI: 10.1161/HYPERTENSIONAHA.110.162446

[11] Hu FB, Willett WC, Li T, et al. Adiposity as compared with physical activity in predicting mortality among women. New England Journal of Medicine. 2004;**351**:2694-2703. DOI: 10.1056/NEJMoa042135

[12] Kodama S, Saito K, Tanaka S, et al. Cardiorespiratory fitness as a quantitative predictor of all-cause mortality and cardiovascular events in healthy men and women: A meta-analysis. The Journal of the American Medical Association. 2009;**301**:2024-2035. DOI: 10.1001/jama.2009.681

[13] Myers J, McAuley P, Lavie CJ, et al. Physical activity and cardiorespiratory fitness as major markers of cardiovascular risk: Their independent and interwoven importance to health status. Progress in Cardiovascular Diseases. 2015;**57**:306-314. DOI: 10.1016/j.pcad.2014.09.011

[14] Myers J, Kaykha A, George S, et al. Fitness versus physical activity patterns in predicting mortality in men. American Journal of Medicine. 2004;**117**:912-918. DOI: 10.1016/j.amjmed.2004.06.047

[15] Xiao J. Physical exercise for human health. Advances in Experimental Medicine and Biology. 2020;**1228**:453-455. DOI: 10.1007/978-981-15-1792-1

[16] Garber CE, Blissmer B, Deschenes MR, et al. Quantity and quality of exercise for developing and maintaining cardiorespiratory, musculoskeletal, and neuromotor fitness in apparently healthy adults. Medicine & Science in Sports & Exercise. 2012;**43**:1334-1359. DOI: 10.1249/MSS.0b013e318213fefb

[17] Vanhees L, Rauch B, Piepoli M, et al. Importance of characteristics and modalities of physical activity and exercise in the management of cardiovascular health in individuals with cardiovascular disease (part III). European Journal of Preventive Cardiology. 2012;**19**:1333-1356. DOI: 10.1177/2047487312437063

[18] Moore DR, Burd NA. Exercise intensity matters for both young and old muscles. Journal of Physiology. 2009;**1587**:511-513. DOI: 10.1113/jphysiol.2008.166744

[19] Wu NN, Tian H, Chen P, et al. Physical exercise and selective autophagy: Benefit and risk on cardiovascular health. Cell. 2019;**8**:1436. DOI: 10.3390/cells8111436

[20] Piercy KL, Troiano RP, Ballard RM, et al. The physical activity guidelines for Americans. The Journal of the American Medical Association. 2018;**320**:2020-2028. DOI: 10.1001/jama.2018.14854

[21] Macdonald JR. Potential causes and mechanisms of postexercise hypotension [thesis]. Macdougall Duncan Journal. 2000;**4**:57-73

[22] Evaristo S, Moreira C, Lopes L, et al. Muscular fitness and cardiorespiratory fitness are associated with health-related quality of life: Results from labmed physical activity study. Journal of Exercise Science and Fitness. 2019;**17**:55-61. DOI: 10.1016/j.jesf.2019.01.002

[23] Williams MA, Haskell WL, Ades PA, et al. Resistance exercise in individuals with and without cardiovascular disease: 2007 update: A scientific statement from the American Heart Association Council on clinical cardiology and council on nutrition, physical activity, and metabolism. Circulation. 2015;**116**:572-584. DOI: 10.1161/CIRCULATIONAHA.107.185214

[24] Mann S, Beedie C, Jimenez A. Differential effects of aerobic exercise, resistance training and combined exercise modalities on cholesterol and the lipid profile: Review, synthesis and recommendations. Sports Medicine. 2014;**44**:221, 10.1007/s40279-013-0110-5-221

[25] Ekblom-Bak E, Ekblom B, Vikstrom M, et al. The importance of non-exercise physical activity for cardiovascular health and longevity. British Journal of Sports Medicine. 2014;**48**:233, 10.1136/bjsports-2012-092038

[26] Buttar HS, Li T, Ravi N. Prevention of cardiovascular diseases: Role of exercise, dietary interventions, obesity and smoking cessation. Experimental & Clinical Cardiology. 2005;**10**:229-249

[27] Glass CK, Witztum JL. Atherosclerosis: The road ahead. Cell. 2001;**104**:503-516. DOI: 10.1016/S0092-8674(01)00238-0

[28] Avins AL. Hypertriglyceridemia and atherosclerosis. Annals of Internal Medicine. 1998;**128**:73-74. DOI: 10.7326/0003-4819-128-1-199801010-00023

[29] Falk E. Pathogenesis of atherosclerosis. Journal of the American College of Cardiology. 2006;**47**:C7-12. DOI: 10.1016/j.jacc.2005.09.068

[30] Wood G, Murrell A, Touw T, et al. HIIT is not superior to MICT in altering blood lipids: A systematic review and meta-analysis. BMJ Open Sport & Exercise Medicine. 2019;**5**:e000647. DOI: 10.1136/bmjsem-2019-000647

[31] Leon AS, Sanchez OA. Response of blood lipids to exercise training alone or combined with dietary intervention. Medicine Science Sports Exercise. 2001;**33**:S502. DOI: 10.1097/00005768-200106001-00021

[32] Kraus WE, Houmard JA, Duscha BD, et al. Effects of the amount and intensity of exercise on plasma lipoproteins. The New England Journal of Medicine. 2002;**347**:1483-1492. DOI: 10.1097/00005768-200106001-00021

[33] Donovan GO, Owen A, Bird SR, et al. Changes in cardiorespiratory fitness and coronary heart disease risk factors following 24 wk of moderate- or high-intensity exercise of equal energy cost. Journal of Applied Physiology. 2005;**98**:1619-1625. DOI: 10.1152/japplphysiol.01310.2004

[34] Horowitz JF, Klein S. Lipid metabolism during endurance exercise. American Journal of Clinical Nutrition. 2000;**72**:558S-563S. DOI: 10.1093/ajcn/72.2.558S

[35] Ferguson MA, Alderson NL, Trost SG, et al. Effects of four different single exercise sessions on lipids, lipoproteins, and lipoprotein lipase. Journal of Applied Physiology. 1998;**85**:1169-1174. DOI: 10.1007/s004210050433

[36] Gast KB, Nathanja T, Theo S, et al. Insulin resistance and risk of incident cardiovascular events in adults without diabetes: Meta-analysis. PLoS One. 2012;7:e52036. DOI: 10.1371/journal.pone.0052036

[37] Defronzo RA, Banerji MA, Bray GA, et al. Determinants of glucose tolerance in impaired glucose tolerance at baseline in the actos now for prevention of diabetes (ACT NOW) study. Diabetologia. 2010;**53**:435-445. DOI: 10.1007/s00125-009-1614-2

[38] Cullen MT, Brice E, Kahn CRK. Critical nodes in signalling pathways: Insights into insulin action. Nature Reviews Molecular Cell Biology. 2006;7:85. DOI: 10.1038/nrm1837

[39] Hirosumi J, Tuncman G, Chang L, et al. A central role for JNK in obesity and insulin resistance. Nature. 2002;**420**:333-336. DOI: 10.1038/nature01137

[40] Wilkes JJ, Hevener A, Olefsky J. Chronic endothelin-1 treatment leads to insulin resistance in vivo. Diabetes. 2003;**52**:1904. DOI: 10.2337/diabetes.52.8.1904

[41] Dominique H, Dorien, et al. Impact of endurance exercise training in the fasted state on muscle biochemistry and metabolism in healthy subjects: Can these effects be of particular clinical benefit to type2 diabetes mellitus and insulin-resistant patients? Sports Medicine. 2016;**47**:1-14. DOI: 10.1007/s40279-016-0594-x

[42] Boulé NG, Kenny GP, Haddad E, et al. Meta-analysis of the effect

of structured exercise training on cardiorespiratory fitness in type 2 diabetes mellitus. Diabetologia. 2003;**46**:1071-1081. DOI: 10.1007/s00125-003-1160-2

[43] Msc DU. Physical activity advice only or structured exercise training and association with HbA1c levels in type 2 diabetes: A systematic review and meta-analysis. JAMA. 2011;**305**:1790. DOI: 10.1001/jama.2011.576

[44] Umpierre D, Ribeiro P, Schaan BD, et al. Volume of supervised exercise training impacts glycaemic control in patients with type 2 diabetes: A systematic review with meta-regression analysis. Diabetologia. 2013;**56**:242-251. DOI: 10.1007/s00125-012-2774-z

[45] Church TS et al. Effects of aerobic and resistance training on Hemoglobin A1cLevels in patients with type 2 diabetes. JAMA. 2010;**304**:2253-2262. DOI: 10.1001/jama.2010.1710

[46] Sylow L et al. Exercise-stimulated glucose uptake—Regulation and implications for glycaemic control. Nature Reviews Endocrinology. 2016;**13**:133-148. DOI: 10.1038/nrendo.2016.162

[47] Hespel P et al. Important role of insulin and flow in stimulating glucose uptake in contracting skeletal muscle. Diabetes. 1995;**44**(2):210-215

[48] Kennedy JW et al. Acute exercise induces GLUT4 translocation in skeletal muscle of normal human subjects and subjects with type 2 diabetes. Diabetes. 1999;**48**(5):1192-1197

[49] Williams B et al. 2018 ESC/ESH guidelines for the management of arterial hypertension. Journal of Hypertension. 2018;**36**(12):2284-2309

[50] Acelajado MC, Calhoun DA, Oparil S. Pathogenesis of hypertension. Pathogenesis of Hypertension. 2012. DOI: 10.1016/B978-1-4377-2766-1.00002-8

[51] Donna K, Arnett, et al. ACC/AHA guideline on the primary prevention of cardiovascular disease. Circulation. 2019;**140**:e596-e646. DOI: 10.1161/CIR.0000000000000678

[52] Mancia G, Fagard R, Narkiewicz K, et al. 2013 ESH/ESC practice guidelines for the management of arterial hypertension. Blood Pressure. 2014;**25**:3-16. DOI: 10.3109/08037051.2014.868629

[53] Dasgupta K, Quinn RR, Zarnke KB, et al. The 2014 Canadian hypertension education program recommendations for blood pressure measurement, diagnosis, assessment of risk, prevention, and treatment of hypertension. Canadian Journal of Cardiology. 2014;**30**:485-501. DOI: 10.1016/j.cjca.2014.02.002

[54] Johnson BT, MacDonald HV, Bruneau ML, et al. Methodological quality of meta-analyses on the blood pressure response to exercise: A review. Journal of Hypertension. 2014;**32**(4). DOI: 10.1097/HJH.0000000000000097

[55] Kenney MJ, Seals DR. Key features, mechanisms, and clinical significance. Hypertension. 1993;**22**:653-664. DOI: 10.1161/01.hyp.22.5.653

[56] Pescatello LS, MacDonald HV, Lamberti L, et al. Exercise for hypertension: A prescription update integrating existing recommendations with emerging research. Current Hypertension Reports. 2015;**17**:87. DOI: 10.1007/s11906-015-0600-y

[57] Liu S, Goodman J, Nolan R, et al. Blood pressure responses to acute and chronic exercise are related in prehypertension. Medicine & Science in Sports & Exercise. 2012;**44**:1644-1652. DOI: 10.1249/MSS.0b013e31825408fb

[58] Eicher JD, Maresh CM, Tsongalis GJ, et al. The additive blood pressure lowering effects of exercise intensity on post-exercise hypotension. American Heart Journal. 2010;**160**:513-520. DOI: 10.1016/j.ahj.2010.06.005

[59] Dimeo F, Pagonas N, Seibert F, et al. Aerobic exercise reduces blood pressure in resistant hypertension. Hypertension. 2012;**60**:653-658. DOI: 10.1161/HYPERTENSIONAHA.112.197780

[60] Sabbahi A, Arena R, Elokda A, et al. Exercise and hypertension: Uncovering the mechanisms of vascular control. Progress in Cardiovascular Diseases. 2016;**59**:226-234. DOI: 10.1016/j.pcad.2016.09.006

[61] Fisher JP, Paton JF. The sympathetic nervous system and blood pressure in humans: Implications for hypertension. Journal of Human Hypertension. 2012;**26**:463-475. DOI: 10.1038/jhh.2011.66

[62] Fadel PJ, Raven PB. Human investigations into the arterial and cardiopulmonary baroreflexes during exercise. Experimental Physiology. 2011;**97**:39-50. DOI: 10.1113/expphysiol.2011.057554

[63] Laterza MC, Matos LD, Trombetta IC, et al. Exercise training restores baroreflex sensitivity in never-treated hypertensive patients. Hypertension. 2007;**49**:1298-1306. DOI: 10.1161/HYPERTENSIONAHA.106.085548

[64] Green DJ, Maiorana A, O'Driscoll G, et al. Effect of exercise training on endothelium-derived nitric oxide function in humans. The Journal of Physiology. 2004;**561**:1-25. DOI: 10.1113/jphysiol.2004.068197

[65] Van Guilder GP, Westby CM, Greiner JJ, et al. Endothelin-1 vasoconstrictor tone increases with age in healthy men but can be reduced by regular aerobic exercise. Hypertension. 2007;**50**:403-409. DOI: 10.1161/HYPERTENSIONAHA

[66] Maiorana A, O'Driscoll G, Taylor R, et al. Exercise and the nitric oxide vasodilator system. Sports Medicine. 2003;**33**:1013-1035. DOI: 10.2165/00007256-200333140-00001

[67] Pedralli ML, Marschner RA, Kollet DP, et al. Different exercise training modalities produce similar endothelial function improvements in individuals with prehypertension or hypertension: A randomized clinical trial exercise, endothelium and blood pressure. Scientific Reports. 2020;**10**:7628. DOI: 10.1038/s41598-020-64365-x

[68] Maeda S, Tanabe T, Miyauchi T, et al. Aerobic exercise training reduces plasma endothelin-1 concentration in older women. Journal of Applied Physiology. 2003;**95**:336-341. DOI: 10.1152/japplphysiol.01016.2002

[69] Tanaka H, Dinenno FA, Monahan KD, et al. Aging, habitual exercise, and dynamic arterial compliance. Circulation. 2000;**102**:1270-1275. DOI: 10.1161/01.cir.102.11.1270

[70] Ferrier KE, Waddell TK, Gatzka CD, et al. Aerobic exercise training does not modify large-artery compliance in isolated systolic hypertension. Hypertension. 2001;**38**:222-226. DOI: 10.1161/01.hyp.38.2.222

[71] Aizawa K, Petrella RJ. Acute and chronic impact of dynamic exercise on arterial stiffness in older hypertensives. The Open Cardiovascular Medicine Journal. 2008;**2**:3-8. DOI: 10.2174/1874192400802010003

[72] Stewart KJ, Bacher AC, Turner KL, et al. Effect of exercise on blood pressure in older persons: A randomized controlled trial. Archives of Internal Medicine. 2005;**14**:13-14. DOI: 10.1001/archinte.165.7.756

[73] Tanaka H, Monahan KD, Seals DR. Age-predicted maximal heart rate revisited. Journal of the American College of Cardiology. 2001;**37**:153-156. DOI: 10.1016/s0735-1097(00)01054-8

[74] Valentini M, Parati G. Variables influencing heart rate. Progress in Cardiovascular Diseases. 2009;**52**:11-19. DOI: 10.1016/j.pcad.2009.05.004

[75] Perret-Guillaume C, Joly L, Benetos A. Heart rate as a risk factor for cardiovascular disease. Progress in Cardiovascular Diseases. 2009;**52**:6-10. DOI: 10.1016/j.pcad.2009.05.003

[76] Vikhorev PG, Vikhoreva NN. Cardiomyopathies and related changes in contractility of human heart muscle. International Journal of Molecular Sciences. 2018;**19**:2234. DOI: 10.3390/ijms19082234

[77] MacLeod KT. Recent advances in understanding cardiac contractility in health and disease. F1000Research. 2016;**5**. DOI: 10.12688/f1000research.8661.1

[78] Tarazi RC, Levy MN. Cardiac responses to increased afterload. State-of-the-art review. Hypertension. 1982;**4**:8-18. DOI: 10.1161/01.HYP.4.3.8

[79] Gewillig M, Brown SC, Eyskens B, et al. The fontan circulation: Who controls cardiac output? Interactive Cardiovascular and Thoracic Surgery. 2010;**10**:428-433. DOI: 10.1510/icvts.2009.218594

[80] Raghuveer G, Hartz J, Lubans DR, et al. Cardiorespiratory fitness in youth: An important marker of health: A scientific statement from the american heart association. Circulation. 2020;**142**:e101-e118. DOI: 10.1161/CIR.0000000000000866

[81] Lang JJ, Wolfe Phillips E, Orpana HM, et al. Field-based measurement of cardiorespiratory fitness to evaluate physical activity interventions. Bulletin of the World Health Organization. 2018;**96**:794. DOI: 10.2471/BLT.18.213728

[82] Cao M, Quan M, Zhuang J. Effect of high-intensity interval training versus moderate-intensity continuous training on cardiorespiratory fitness in children and adolescents: A meta-analysis. International Journal of Environmental Research and Public Health. 2019;**16**:1533. DOI: 10.3390/ijerph16091533

[83] Fernández R, Lvarez B, Ferri M, et al. Pilates method improves cardiorespiratory fitness: A systematic review and meta-analysis. Journal of Clinical Medicine. 2019;**8**:1761. DOI: 10.3390/jcm8111761

[84] Gupta S, Rohatgi A, Ayers CR, et al. Cardiorespiratory fitness and classification of risk of cardiovascular disease mortality. Circulation. 2011;**123**:1377-1383. DOI: 10.1161/CIRCULATIONAHA.110.003236

[85] Posnakidis G, Aphamis G, Giannaki CD, et al. High-intensity functional training improves cardiorespiratory fitness and neuromuscular performance without inflammation or muscle damage. Journal of Strength and Conditioning Research. 2022;**36**:615-623. DOI: 10.1519/JSC.0000000000003516

[86] Liu J, Zhu L, Su Y. Comparative effectiveness of high-intensity interval

training and moderate-intensity continuous training for cardiometabolic risk factors and cardiorespiratory fitness in childhood obesity: A meta-analysis of randomized controlled trials. Frontiers in Physiology. 2020;**11**:214. DOI: 10.3389/fphys.2020.00214

[87] Drzyzga CJ, Bahls M, Ittermann T, et al. Lower cardiorespiratory fitness is associated with right ventricular geometry and function—The sedentary's heart: SHIP. Journal of the American Heart Association. 2021;**10**:e021116. DOI: 10.1161/JAHA.120.021116

[88] Tuan SH, Li CH, Sun SF, et al. Comparison of cardiorespiratory fitness between preschool children with normal and excess body adipose—An observational study. PLoS One. 2019;**14**:e0223907. DOI: 10.1371/journal.pone.0223907

[89] Fels I, Hartman E, Bosker RJ, et al. Effects of aerobic exercise and cognitively engaging exercise on cardiorespiratory fitness and motor skills in primary school children: A cluster randomized controlled trial. Journal of Sports Sciences. 2020;**38**:1975-1983. DOI: 10.1080/02640414.2020.17654641-9

[90] Murias JM, Kowalchuk JM, Paterson DH. Mechanisms for increases in V˙O2max with endurance training in older and young women. Medicine & Science in Sports & Exercise. 2010;**42**:1891-1898. DOI: 10.1249/MSS.0b013e3181dd0bba

[91] García HA, Alonso M, Ramírez VR, et al. Effects of exercise intervention on health-related physical fitness and blood pressure in preschool children: A systematic review and meta-analysis of randomized controlled trials. Sports Medicine. 2020;**50**:187-203. DOI: 10.1007/s40279-019-01191-w

[92] Bauer N, Sperlich B, Holmberg HC, et al. Effects of high-intensity interval training in school on the physical performance and health of children and adolescents: A systematic review with meta-analysis. Sports Medicine—Open. 2022;**8**:50. DOI: 10.1186/s40798-022-00437-8

[93] Engel FA, Ackermann A, Chtourou H, et al. High-intensity interval training performed by young athletes: A systematic review and meta-analysis. Frontiers in Physiology. 2018;**9**:1012. DOI: 10.3389/fphys.2018.01012

[94] Wen D, Utesch T, Wu J, et al. Effects of different protocols of high intensity interval training for VO2max improvements in adults: A meta-analysis of randomised controlled trials. Journal of Science and Medicine in Sport. 2019;**22**:941-947. DOI: 10.1016/j.jsams.2019.01.013

[95] Baar K. Training for endurance and strength: Lessons from cell signaling. Medicine & Science in Sports & Exercise. 2006;**38**:1939-1944. DOI: 10.1249/01.mss.0000233799.62153.19

[96] Fisher J, Steele J, Smith D. High- and low-load resistance training: Interpretation and practical application of current research findings. Sports Medicine. 2017;**47**:393-400. DOI: 10.1007/s40279-016-0602-1

[97] Paoli A, Gentil P, Moro T, et al. Resistance training with single vs. multi-joint exercises at equal total load volume: Effects on body composition, cardiorespiratory fitness, and muscle strength. Frontiers in Physiology. 2017;**8**:1-6. DOI: 10.3389/fphys.2017.01105

[98] Birkett ST, Nichols S, Sawrey R, et al. The effects of low-volume high-intensity interval training and circuit training

on maximal oxygen uptake. Sport Sciences for Health. 2019;**15**:443-451. DOI: 10.1007/s11332-019-00552-2

[99] Poon E, Wongpipit W, Ho R, et al. Interval training versus moderate-intensity continuous training for cardiorespiratory fitness improvements in middle-aged and older adults: A systematic review and meta-analysis. Journal of Sports Sciences. 2021;**39**:1996-2005. DOI: 10.1080/02640414.2021.1912453

[100] Ramos CD, Andreu CL, Carrasco PM, et al. Effects of circuit resistance training on body composition, strength, and cardiorespiratory fitness in middle-aged and older women: A systematic review and meta-analysis. Journal of Aging and Physical Activity. 2021;**1**:1-14. DOI: 10.1123/japa.2021-0204

[101] Ballesta GI, Martínez GI, Ramos CJ, et al. High-intensity interval circuit training versus moderate-intensity continuous training on cardiorespiratory fitness in middle-aged and older women: A randomized controlled trial. International Journal of Environmental Research and Public Health. 2020;**17**:1805. DOI: 10.3390/ijerph17051805

[102] Bherer L, Langeard A, Kaushal N, et al. Physical exercise training effect and mediation through cardiorespiratory fitness on dual-task performances differ in younger–old and older–old adults. The Journals of Gerontology: Series B. 2021;**76**:219-228. DOI: 10.1093/geronb/gbz066

[103] Smith PJ, Blumenthal JA, Hoffman BM, et al. Aerobic exercise and neurocognitive performance: A meta-analytic review of randomized controlled trials. Psychosomatic Medicine. 2010;**72**:239. DOI: 10.1016/j.neubiorev.2017.04.011

[104] Ramos JS, Dalleck LC, Tjonna AE, et al. The impact of high-intensity interval training versus moderate-intensity continuous training on vascular function: A systematic review and meta-analysis. Sports Medicine. 2015;**45**:679-692. DOI: 10.1007/s40279-015-0321-z

[105] Lindsay SG, Banting L, Eime R, et al. The association between social support and physical activity in older adults: A systematic review. International Journal of Behavioral Nutrition and Physical Activity. 2017;**14**:1-21. DOI: 10.1186/s12966-017-0509-8

[106] Heiland EG, Welmer AK, Wang R, et al. Cardiovascular risk factors and the risk of disability in older adults: Variation by age and functional status. Journal of the American Medical Directors Association. 2019;**20**(208-12):e3. DOI: 10.1016/j.jamda.2018.05.013

[107] Wu ZJ, Wang ZY, Gao HE, et al. Impact of high-intensity interval training on cardiorespiratory fitness, body composition, physical fitness, and metabolic parameters in older adults: A meta-analysis of randomized controlled trials. Experimental Gerontology. 2021;**150**:111345. DOI: 10.1016/j.exger.2021.111345

[108] Vincent KR, Braith RW, Feldman RA, et al. Improved cardiorespiratory endurance following 6 months of resistance exercise in elderly men and women. Archives of Internal Medicine. 2002;**162**:673-678. DOI: 10.1001/archinte.162.6.673

[109] Coetsee C, Terblanche E. The effect of three different exercise training modalities on cognitive and physical function in a healthy older population. European Review of Aging and Physical Activity. 2017;**14**:1-10. DOI: 10.1186/s11556-017-0183-5

[110] Garber CE, Blissmer B, Deschenes MR, et al. Quantity and quality of exercise for developing and maintaining cardiorespiratory, musculoskeletal, and neuromotor fitness in apparently healthy adults: Guidance for prescribing exercise. Medicine & Science in Sports & Exercise. 2011;**43**:1334-1359. DOI: 10.1249/MSS.0b013e318213fefb

[111] Pate RR, Pate JR, Neill O. Physical activity guidelines for young children an emerging consensus. Archives of Pediatrics & Adolescent Medicine. 2012;**166**:1095-1096. DOI: 10.3390/cells8111436

[112] Nelson ME, Rejeski WJ, Blair SN, et al. Physical activity and public health in older adults: Recommendation from the American College of Sports Medicine and the American Heart Association. Medicine Science Sports Exercise. 2007;**39**:1435-1445. DOI: 10.1249/mss.0b013e3180616aa2

[113] Franklin BA, Lavie CJ, Squires RW, et al. Exercise-based cardiac rehabilitation and improvements in cardiorespiratory fitness: Implications regarding patient benefit. Mayo Clinic Proceedings. 2013;**88**:431-437. DOI: 10.1016/j.mayocp.2013.03.013

[114] Bernardo BC, Ooi J, Weeks KL, et al. Understanding key mechanisms of exercise-induced cardiac protection to mitigate disease: Current knowledge and emerging concepts. Physiological Reviews. 2018;**98**:419-475. DOI: 10.1152/physrev.00043.2016

[115] Eijsvogels TM, Fernandez AB, Thompson PD. Are there deleterious cardiac effects of acute and chronic endurance exercise? Physiological Reviews. 2016;**96**:99-125. DOI: 10.1152/physrev.00029.2014

[116] Siasos G, Athanasiou D, Terzis G, et al. Acute effects of different types of aerobic exercise on endothelial function and arterial stiffness. European Journal of Preventive Cardiology. 2016;**23**:1565-1572. DOI: 10.1177/2047487316647185

[117] Way KL, Sultana RN, Sabag A, et al. The effect of high intensity interval training versus moderate intensity continuous training on arterial stiffness and 24h blood pressure responses: A systematic review and meta-analysis. Journal of Science and Medicine in Sport. 2019;**22**:385-391. DOI: 10.1016/j.jsams.2018.09.228

[118] O'Donovan G, Blazevich AJ, Boreham C, et al. The ABC of physical activity for health: A consensus statement from the British Association of Sport and Exercise Sciences. Journal of Sports Sciences. 2010;**28**:573-591. DOI: 10.1080/02640411003671212

[119] Izquierdo M, Morley JE, Anker SD. International exercise recommendations in older adults (ICFSR): Expert consensus guidelines. Journal of Nutrition, Health & Aging. 2021;**25**:824-853. DOI: 10.1007/s12603-021-1665-8

[120] Myers J, Kokkinos P, Nyelin E. Physical activity, cardiorespiratory fitness, and the metabolic syndrome. Nutrients. 2019;**11**:1652. DOI: 10.3390/nu11071652

[121] Kraemer WJ, Adams K, Farelli E, et al. American College of Sports Medicine position stand. Progression models in resistance training for healthy adults. Medicine Science Sports Exercise. 2009;**41**:687-708. DOI: 10.1097/00005768-200202000-00027

[122] López MS, Sánchez M, Solera M, et al. Physical activity, fitness, and metabolic syndrome in young adults. Sport Nutrition and Exercise Metabolism. 2013;**23**:312-321. DOI: 10.1038/ijo.2013.89

[123] Verrill DE, Ribisl PM. Resistive exercise training in cardiac rehabilitation. Sports Medicine. 1996;**21**:347-383. DOI: 10.2165/00007256-199621050-00004

[124] Candow DG, Burke DG. Effect of short-term equal-volume resistance training with different workout frequency on muscle mass and strength in untrained men and women. Journal of Strength and Conditioning Research. 2007;**21**:204-207. DOI: 10.1519/R-19785.1

[125] Schoenfeld BJ, Ogborn D, Krieger JW. Effects of resistance training frequency on measures of muscle hypertrophy: A systematic review and meta-analysis. Sports Medicine. 2016;**46**:1689-1697. DOI: 10.1007/s40279-016-0543-8

[126] Grgic J, Schoenfeld BJ, Davies TB, et al. Effect of resistance training frequency on gains in muscular strength: A systematic review and meta-analysis. Sports Medicine. 2018;**48**:1207-1220. DOI: 10.1007/s40279-018-0872-x

[127] Kraemer WJ, Ratamess NA. Fundamentals of resistance training: Progression and exercise prescription. Medicine Science Sports Exercise. 2004;**36**:674-688. DOI: 10.1249/01.MSS.0000121945.36635.61

[128] García A, Sánchez M, Martínez V. Effects of aerobic plus resistance exercise on body composition related variables in pediatric obesity: A systematic review and meta-analysis of randomized controlled trials. Pediatric Exercise Science. 2015;**27**:431-440. DOI: 10.1123/pes.2014-0132

[129] Vinetti G, Mozzini C, Desenzani P, et al. Supervised exercise training reduces oxidative stress and cardiometabolic risk in adults with type 2 diabetes: A randomized controlled trial. Scientific Reports. 2015;**5**:9238. DOI: 10.1038/srep09238

[130] Kosek DJ, Kim JS, Petrella JK, et al. Efficacy of 3 days/wk resistance training on myofiber hypertrophy and myogenic mechanisms in young vs. older adults. Journal of Applied Physiology. 2006;**101**:531-544. DOI: 10.1152/japplphysiol.01474.2005

[131] Nunes JP, Grgic J, Cunha PM, et al. What influence does resistance exercise order have on muscular strength gains and muscle hypertrophy? A systematic review and meta-analysis. European Journal Sport Science. 2021;**21**:149-157. DOI: 10.1080/17461391.2020.1733672

[132] Izquierdo M, Merchant RA, Morley JE, et al. International exercise recommendations in older adults (ICFSR): Expert consensus guidelines. Journal Nutrition Health Aging. 2021;**25**:824-853. DOI: 10.1007/s12603-021-1665-8

[133] Schroeder EC, Franke WD, Sharp RL, et al. Comparative effectiveness of aerobic, resistance, and combined training on cardiovascular disease risk factors: A randomized controlled trial. PLoS One. 2019;**14**(1):e0210292. DOI: 10.1371/journal.pone.0210292

[134] Alberga AS, Prud D, Sigal RJ, et al. Effects of aerobic training, resistance training, or both on cardiorespiratory and musculoskeletal fitness in adolescents with obesity: The HEARTY trial. Applied Physiology Nutrition and Metabolism. 2016;**41**:255-265. DOI: 10.1139/apnm-2015-0413

[135] Brellenthin AG, Lanningham LM, Kohut ML, et al. Comparison of the cardiovascular benefits of resistance, aerobic, and combined exercise (CardioRACE): Rationale, design, and methods. American Heart Journal. 2019;**217**:101-111. DOI: 10.1016/j.ahj.2019.08.00828

Chapter 2

Assessment of Exercise Capacity: A Key Element in Pulmonary Rehabilitation

Paraschiva Postolache, Ștefan Săndulache, Constantin Ghimuș and Alexandru Nechifor

Abstract

Pulmonary rehabilitation (PR) is an extremely effective treatment for people with chronic lung disease, including post-COVID-19, which is still underused worldwide. The capacity for effort and its increase through physical training is a key element that underlies the PR programs being recognized by all specialists in the field in the guides of the American Thoracic Society (ATS)/European Respiratory Society (ERS), American Association of Cardiovascular and Pulmonary Rehabilitation (AACVPR), American College of Sports Medicine (ACSM), Global Initiative for Chronic Obstructive Lung Disease (GOLD), etc. The evaluation helps to determine the factors that limit it (ventilators, cardiovascular and muscular factors, etc.), to prescribe the intensity of training, to detect the contraindications of PR, and to evaluate the effectiveness of the rehabilitation program (improving exercise capacity, reducing exercise dyspnea, etc.). In clinical practice, we use two types of investigations on exercise capacity: maximal test (cardiopulmonary exertion test) and submaximal test (6-minute walk test). Based on the systematic review of recent literature and our clinical experience, the chapter will highlight issues related to PR, exercise capacity, and physical training (aerobic, endurance, respiratory muscle) in patients with chronic lung disease.

Keywords: pulmonary rehabilitation, COPD, exercise capacity, dyspnea, quality of life

1. Introduction

We decided to start this chapter by challenging the reader with four questions. Sometimes, the answers can be provocative. However, they stimulate scientific and clinical discussion on this topic:

1. **Is pulmonary rehabilitation an effective treatment?**

Answer: Pulmonary rehabilitation (PR) is an extremely effective treatment for people with chronic lung disease, including post-COVID-19, still underused worldwide, being recognized by all specialists in the field of the American Thoracic Society

(ATS), European Respiratory Society (ERS), American Association of Cardiovascular and Pulmonary Rehabilitation (AACVPR), American College of Sports Medicine (ACSM), Global Initiative for Chronic Obstructive Lung Disease (GOLD), etc.

2. **Is it important to assess dyspnea for notice the changes in exercise capacity during pulmonary rehabilitation programs?**

Answer: Yes, dyspnea is a central symptom of a patient with chronic respiratory disease and can be present both at rest and during exertion. Reducing dyspnea is one of the goals of the pulmonary rehabilitation program.

3. **What tests are essential in assessing exercise capacity and prescribing a training program?**

Answer: The 6-minute walk test, cardiopulmonary exercise test, and respiratory muscle strength testing are fundamental.

4. **Is physical training (aerobics, endurance, respiratory muscles, etc.) a guarantee to meet the needs of the patient? How should the training intensity be adapted for the patient to cope with the proposed training intensity?**

Answer: Physical training is an essential component of a PR program. To answer the first question: Yes, the improvement of exercise capacity and muscle strength should be implemented in the daily life of the patient and not only during the PR sessions in specialized centers, to increase their quality of life. We would answer the second question: The intensity of training is determined by the maximum effort capacity obtained in testing, the severity of the condition, the age of the patient, and the severity of comorbidities, using interval and/or continuous training for proper adaptation to training and maximum benefit.

2. Pulmonary rehabilitation: definition, objectives, evaluation

Over the las century, many innovative data and ideas about PR have been accumulated worldwide, as well as the development of an arsenal of techniques for assessing and developing respiratory function. These data and ideas support the progress of modern medicine and the concern about expanding lung disease. With modern industrialization, development of the chemical industry, and urbanization, the human body, and last but not the least, the respiratory system has been exposed to increasingly harmful risk factors.

PR is essential for these patients, being recognized by all specialists. The current definition of PR, according to the Official ATS Workshop Report published on May 2021, is based on the scientifically developed definitions previously developed by PR specialists, which have been published since 1974 and updated in 2006, 2007, 2013, 2015. According to this report, "pulmonary rehabilitation is a comprehensive intervention based on a thorough patient assessment followed by patient-tailored therapies that include, but are not limited to, exercise training, education and behavior change, designed to improve the physical and psychological condition of people with chronic respiratory disease and to promote the ling-term adherence to health-enhancing behaviors" [1–5].

PR is an extremely effective treatment for people with chronic lung disease, including post-COVID-19, which is still underused worldwide. In recent years, new models of PR programs have emerged, which aim to improve access and adopt these methods to current conditions, such as telerehabilitation and low-cost models, useful for PR at home. Comprehensive and thorough assessment of the patient is essential for personalizing the PR program and for effectively addressing its objectives tailored to each patient. The processes of assessing the quality of life provided by PR are important to ensure that any PR service delivers optimal results for patients and health services. The success of these PR models is evaluated by the way of achieving the essential components of the PR programs (**Figure 1**) and the results expected by the patient, such as improving exercise capacity, reducing symptoms, especially dyspnea, fatigue, cough, expectoration, chest pain, anxiety and depression, reducing the number and severity of exacerbations involving hospitalization and improving health-related quality of life [1, 4–9].

The initial assessment of patients for inclusion in the PR program needs:

- History and objective examination for the underlying disease and comorbidities;
- Evaluation of the contraindications that may require not starting the PR program;
- Evaluation of the medication and the therapeutic scheme followed until the moment of inclusion in the PR program;
- Smoking status assessment—modified Fagerström test to assess nicotine addiction [10];
- assessment of nutritional status—body mass index (BMI);
- body composition—evaluated by body-plethysmography, which uses the densitometry of the whole body;
- measuring the strength of peripheral muscles;
- symptomatic assessment of:
    - dyspnea (modified Medical Research Council scale—mMRC for the assessment of resting dyspnea and the Borg scale for the evaluation of exertional dyspnea);

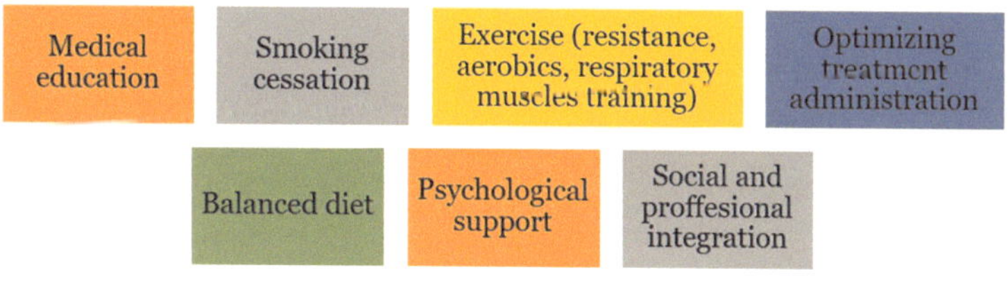

Figure 1.
Pulmonary rehabilitation components [2, 6].

- fatigue Assessment Scale (FAS) [11];
- in patients with asthma, the Asthma Control Test (ACT) questionnaire is also completed;
- in COPD patients, the COPD Assessment Test (CAT) questionnaire is also completed;

- evaluation of the performance of daily activities—the Instrumental Activity of Daily Living (IADL) questionnaire [12, 13];
- quality of life assessment—SF-36 (The 36-Item Short Form Survey) [14];
- evaluation of medical education—Lung Information Needs Questionnaire (LINQ) [15];
- spirometry ± bronchial reversibility test;
- body plethysmography;
- diffusion/transfer through the alveolo-capillary membrane of carbon monoxide (diffusing capacity of lung for carbon monoxide: DLCO / TLCO);
- pulse oscillometry (completes the battery of lung function tests, but is not yet included in the routine assessment);
- electrocardiogram; echocardiography;
- exercise capacity assessment—6-minute walk test (6-minute WT), oximetry test, cardiopulmonary exercise test (CPET);
- chest radiography, chest computed tomography (CT);
- assessment of additional needs (wheelchair, walker, O2, CPAP) [1, 3, 5, 16].

There is no universal program applicable to each patient [17], and the PR team is mentioned in **Figure 2**:

A pulmonary rehabilitation program, in terms of good adherence to the patient's treatment, is effective if:

- a reduction in the decline of lung function is obtained;
- an increase in exercise capacity is obtained (for example, improving the 6-minute WT by 10–25% or reducing the sensation of dyspnea during exercise);
- the quality of life is improved by increasing the degree of independence in carrying out daily activities;
- reduces the feeling of dyspnea, fatigue, depression and/or anxiety, etc.;

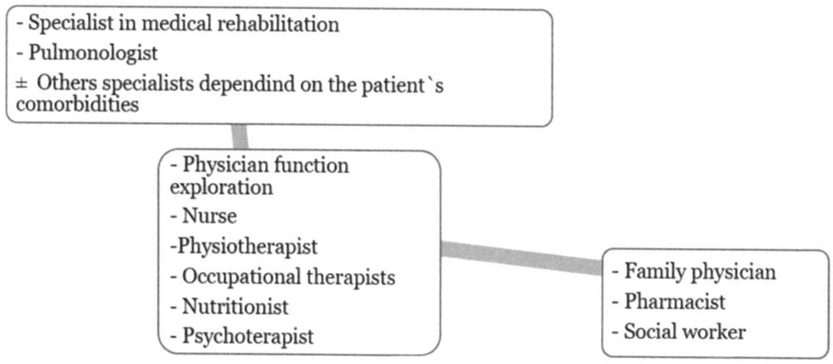

Figure 2.
The team involved in respiratory rehabilitation [1, 2, 16].

- it reduces the number and severity of exacerbations and increases the time until a new exacerbation occurs [18].

3. Dyspnea assessment

Dyspnea is the most common symptom responsible for limiting the exercise capacity of patients with chronic respiratory disease and may be present both at rest and during exercise. The ATS defined dyspnea as: "a term used to describe a subjective experience of respiratory discomfort consisting of qualitatively distinct sensations that may vary in intensity; this subjective experience comes from the interaction of multiple physiological, psychological, social, or environmental factors" [19]. It should be noted that the difficulty in defining, describing, and quantifying dyspnea comes from its subjective nature, due to the involvement of psychological, affective, and cognitive factors.

Reducing dyspnea is one of the goals of the PR program. However, dyspnea is a subjective sensation that is not always related to the severity of the disease. The level of dyspnea is assessed at the beginning and in the end of the PR program, but also during cardiopulmonary exercise test, exercise training sessions, etc. [16].

Various valid and reproducible questionnaires are used to measure dyspnea (**Figure 3**). These must be correlated with other assessment tools, such as respiratory capacity and function.

4. Effort capacity assessment

Effort capacity is the maximum amount of physical effort a patient can withstand. An accurate assessment of exercise capacity requires that the maximum effort be prolonged enough to have a stable (or balanced) effect on circulation and that the patient's response pattern be consistent when the effort is repeated [26].

The roles of effort assessment are represented by the following:

- determining the factors that limit the capacity of effort (ventilator, cardiovascular, muscular);

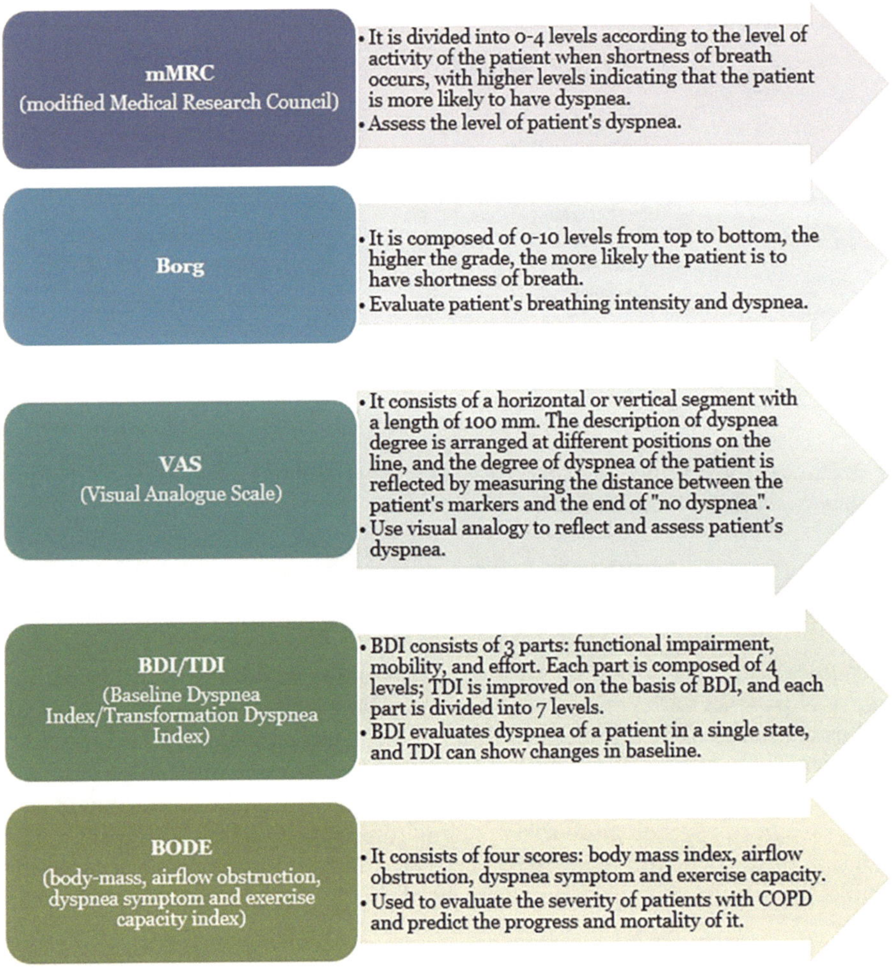

Figure 3.
Assessment of dyspnea [20–25].

- prescribing training intensity;
- detection of contraindications for PR program (e.g., arrhythmia, ischemia, high blood pressure during exercise, etc.);
- evaluation of the effectiveness of the PR program—improving exercise capacity, improving exercise-related dyspnea [27].

In the Respiratory Rehabilitation Clinic of the Rehabilitation Clinical Hospital from Iași, Romania, we routinely use two types of investigations for effort capacity assessment:

- incremental test, maximum: cardiopulmonary exercise test;
- constant submaximal test: 6-minute walk test [16].

4.1 Cardiopulmonary exercise test

At the moment, cardiopulmonary exercise testing (CPET) (**Figure 4**) is the gold standard for exercise testing, being the method that offers the best accuracy and reproductibility, a clearly superior alternative to conventional exercise tests [25].

In addition to classical exercise tests, which are limited to recording the electrocardiogram, pulse, blood oxygen saturation, blood pressure, and subjectively perceived fatigue (Borg scale), during exercise of progressively increasing intensity, CPET involves real-time assessment, at each inhale-exhale cycle, the spirogram and the concentration of the inhaled gases (oxygen and carbon dioxide). Under these conditions, the test allows on overall assessment of the response to physical exertion, integrating the most important physiological systems of the body: respiratory, cardiovascular, musculoskeletal, and neuropsychic.

CPET is a test of maximum effort when the load increases to max VO_2 or limited symptoms VO_2. This type of test has several phases: rest, heating for 3 minutes, than

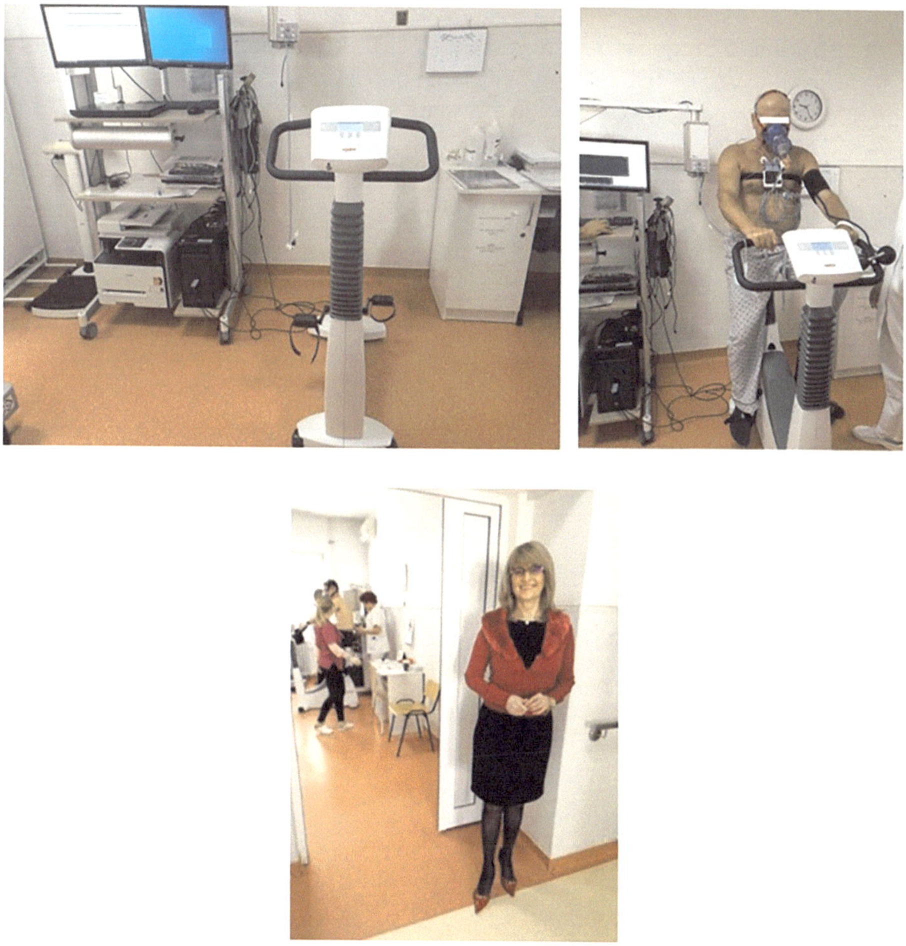

Figure 4.
Cardiopulmonary exercise test. Source photo: Respiratory Rehabilitation Clinic, Rehabilitation Clinical Hospital, Iasi, Romania, Head: Assoc. Prof. Dr. Paraschiva Postolache.

incremental phases in ramp or in steps during 1 minute each. The test can be performed with cycle ergometer or on the treadmill (**Table 1**) [16, 28].

CPET evaluates the following specific and very useful parameters in the PR process:

(a) Maximum oxygen consumption (VO_2 max)

- It is the most accurately parameter used to reflect the maximum exercise capacity, respectively, the maximum level of aerobic metabolism, which can be reached during exercise at the peripheral muscle level (**Figures 5** and **6**).

- Maximum oxygen consumption shows alterations in respiratory pathology, by reducing the level of available peripheral oxygen.

- The periodic evaluation of the maximum oxygen consumption, during PR, allows the objective assessment of the effectiveness of this therapeutic measure, by demonstrating the positive dynamics of VO_2 max.

- It has also a prognostic value, so that in COPD patients, values of VO_2 max in the range of 793–995 ml/min associate an average mortality of 5% at 5 years, while values below 654 ml/min associate a mortality of 60% at 5 years [29, 30].

Cycle ergometer	Treadmill
• Easy to quantify the power of effort;	• Values of maximum oxygen consumption higher by 7–10% can be reached, due to the training of several muscle groups;
• The power of the external effort relatively independent of the patient's weight;	
• Allows ramp protocols, which make it easy to determine the anaerobic threshold;	
• Slightly noisy, which makes it easy to measure blood pressure;	• Better stimulates a patient's usual physical activity;
• The electrocardiogram shows fewer motion artifacts;	
• Lower risk of injury;	• is easier to use for testing low height patients.
• Requires less space.	

Table 1.
Comparative advantages of the exercise test on the cycle ergometer, respective treadmill [28].

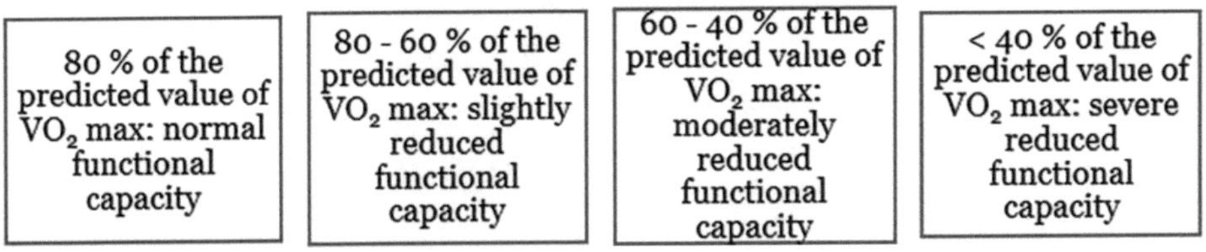

Figure 5.
Limitation of functional capacity according to the value of maximum oxygen consumption [29].

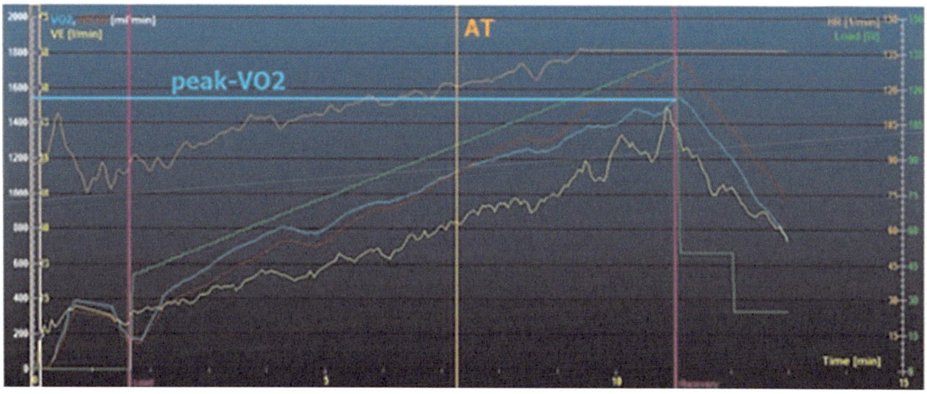

Figure 6.
Graphic determination of maximum oxygen consumption and anaerobic threshold by cardiopulmonary testing. Source photo: Respiratory Rehabilitation Clinic, Rehabilitation Clinical Hospital, Iasi, Romania, Head: Assoc. Prof. Dr. Paraschiva Postolache.

(b) Ventilatory or anaerobic threshold (AT) (**Figure 6**)

- Represents the level of the oxygen consumption at which the cellular metabolism in the peripheral muscles changes from aerobiosis to anaerobiosis, with the increase of lactic acid production, CO_2, and reflex hyperventilation.

- AT is expressed as the value of oxygen consumption at that time or as a percentage of the predicted value of VO_2 max.

- In healthy individuals, AT is in the range of 45–65% of VO_2 max.

- In patients with chronic lung disease, AT is usually reduced to below 40% of VO_2 max (indicating a limitation of tissue oxygen supply).

- Anaerobic threshold is an essential parameter for establishing the optimal level of exercise intensity in PR programs.

- Both at the beginning of the PR program and during it, it is recommended to keep a level of intensity below the anaerobic threshold, the recommended physical exercise being aerobic [29].

(c) Minute ventilation (VE)

- CPET measures ventilation per minute, breath by breath, but also the dynamics of current volume and respiratory rate during exertion, which defines the ventilatory strategy [29].

(d) Inspiratory capacity

- It can be evaluated periodically during CPET, by forced inspiration maneuvers and allows the quantification of dynamic hyperinflation [29].

(e) Ventilation efficiency: slope of the VE/VCO_2 ratio (ventilation/volume of CO_2 produced) at the level of the anaerobic threshold.

- It is the volume of air ventilated in 1 minute, needed to remove 1 liter of CO_2.

- In patients with chronic obstructive respiratory disease, the ratio of VE/VCO_2 has abnormally high values, signifying the alteration of the ventilatory efficiency, as an effect of the increase of the pulmonary dead space and of the alteration of the ventilation/infusion ratio [29, 30].

4.2 The 6-minute walk test

The 6-minute walk test (6MWT) (**Figure 7**, **Tables 2** and **3**) is a constant and submaximal load exercise test (unlike CPET, which is performed at an increasing, incremental load). It is also part of the BODE prognostic index.

As a way of doing things, 6MWT involves:

- The patient, who travels a distance on flat ground for 6 minutes; the number of laps is multiplied by the distance.

- The walking corridor must have an acceptable distance of 30–50 meters.

- The following are evaluated during the test: heart rate, blood pressure, blood saturation, degree of dyspnea (both initially and at the end of the test), and the distance expressed in meters.

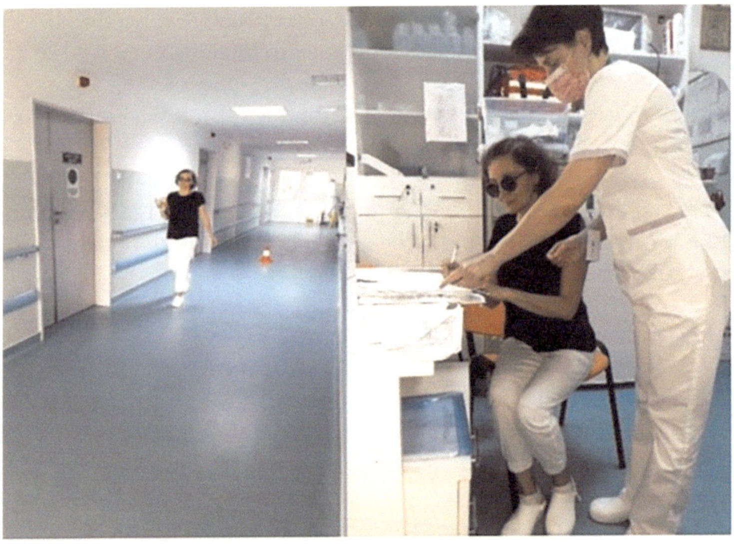

Figure 7.
6-minute walk test. Source photo: Respiratory Rehabilitation Clinic, Rehabilitation Clinical Hospital, Iasi, Romania, Head: Assoc. Prof. Dr. Paraschiva Postolache.

Indications	Contraindications	Test interruption
• Assessment of functional status and disability in COPD, pulmonary fibrosis, cystic fibrosis, pulmonary vascular disease, heart failure;	• Recent myocardial infarction (1 month);	• Chest pain;
		• Intolerable dyspnea;
	• Unstable angina	• Vertigo;
	• Episode of respiratory decompensation with acidosis;	• Extreme weakness;
• Measuring the response to various interventions (pre- and post-treatment comparisons); lung resections, lung rehabilitation, lung transplantation, lung volume reduction surgery, vasodilator treatment in pulmonary hypertension;		• Desaturation <85%;
	• Developmental thrombophlebitis and/ or recent pulmonary embolism;	
		• Tachycardia >80% of the theoretical maximum heart rate (calculated according to the formula: 220—age in years);
	• Acute pericarditis;	
	• Hypertensive emergency;	
	• Bronchospasm crisis;	
	• Fever;	
• Prediction of COPD mortality and morbidity, pulmonary hypertension, pulmonary fibrosis, heart failure;	• Resting tachycardia (> 120/minute) (relative contraindication);	
		• At the express request of the patient.
		• Blood pressure >180/100 at rest (relative contraindication).
• Titration of oxygen flow at exertion.		

Table 2.
Indications, contraindications and limitation of 6MWT [16, 31, 32].

- The patient must walk as far as possible in 6 minutes, walking at his own rhythm, sustained, between the two ends of the aisle, marked with two cones, without running. The patient can stop to rest during the 6 minutes, but must resume walking as soon as possible, the test not lasting with rest time.

- 6MWT results can be expressed as absolute value, percentage of initial value, or percentage of predicted value [16, 31].

Advantage	Disadvantage
• Simple;	• Depends on the motivation of the patient and/or the supervisor;
• Cheap;	
• Good reproducibility (if the standard protocol is followed);	
• Correlates with the prognosis;	• Measures a single variable (distance traveled);
• Can be applied to all patients (regardless of age, level of readiness, degree of respiratory failure);	
	• More difficult to standardize and less reproducible than the maximum effort tests;
• Is a very useful tool in PR programs—it must be done before and after the end of the program, in order to highlight the increase of the distance traveled, with a direct impact in increasing the quality of life.	
	• Does not allow the detection of the causes of the effort limitation.

Table 3.
Advantages and disadvantages 6MWT [31, 33, 34].

Because there are different practices regarding the actual conduct of the test, leading to variable and hard-to-compare results, the international ATS guideline has established clear rules for 6MWT standardization [31, 33].

The following predictable equation, recommended for COPD patients, was used to interpret the results:

- For men: test value (m) = 867 - (5.71 × age) + (1.03 × height)
- For women: test value (m) = 525 – (2.86 × age) + (2.71 × height) – (6.22 × BMI, kg/m^2) [31, 32].

The 6-minute walk test *is considered positive* for an improvement of at least 54 meters compared with the initial assessment [7, 16].

Dosed physical training is one of the most important components of physical therapy and PR programs. The exercise plan is individualized for each patient according to the underlying disease and the degree of severity, age, sex, associated diseases, training methods, duration, pace, intensity of effort, motivation, and choice of the patient [35–38].

Exercise will address different muscle groups:

- to increase the endurance of the muscles of the lower limbs, it is recommended to walk on the treadmill, pedal to the cycle ergometer (**Figure 8**) or to counteract some weights. Exercises should also be performed by people immobilized in a sitting or supine position for limb movement, increased flexibility and decreased joint stiffness, the exercises being focused on stretching, coordination, and attention;

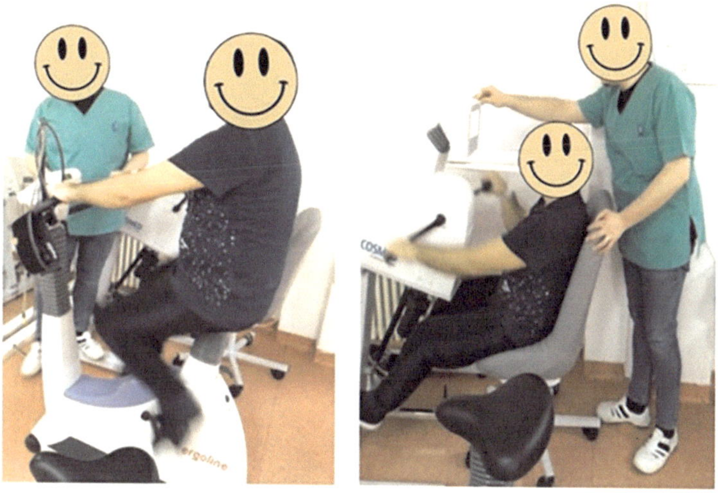

Figure 8.
Physical training dosed on the cycle ergometer for the lower and upper train. Source photo: Respiratory Rehabilitation Clinic, Rehabilitation Clinical Hospital, Iasi, Romania, Head: Assoc. Prof. Dr. Paraschiva Postolache.

- to increase the endurance of the muscles of the upper limbs, the patients will perform exercises with weights or stretching;
- for the chest muscles, stretching, swimming, training on the cycle ergometer or on the treadmill are recommended;
- gymnastics for the neck and head muscles;
- breathing techniques (abdominal breathing, etc.) (**Figure 9**) [26, 35, 36].

4.3 Respiratory muscle assessment

Respiratory muscle training is a valuable method that provides additional PR benefits, improving both muscle strength and endurance, with clinical benefits in

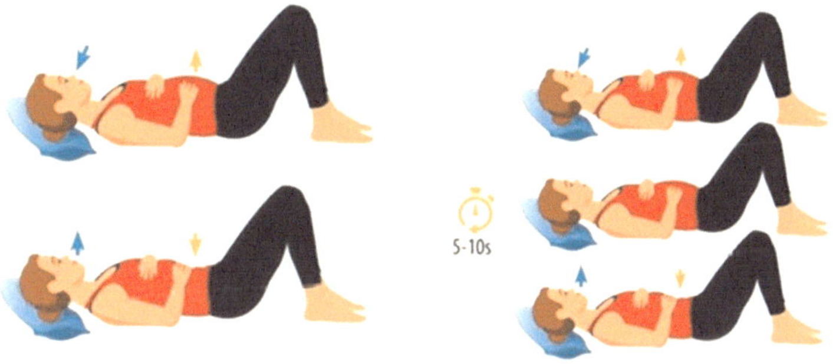

Figure 9.
Basic position in diaphragmatic breathing without and with apnea. Source photo: Material written under the guidance of Assoc. Prof. Dr. Paraschiva Postolache and Physiotherapist Liliana Chelariu, Pulmonary Rehabilitation Clinic, Rehabilitation Clinical Hospital, Iaşi, RO-BRIM-15-2020-V2-exercitii_digital 06.2020.

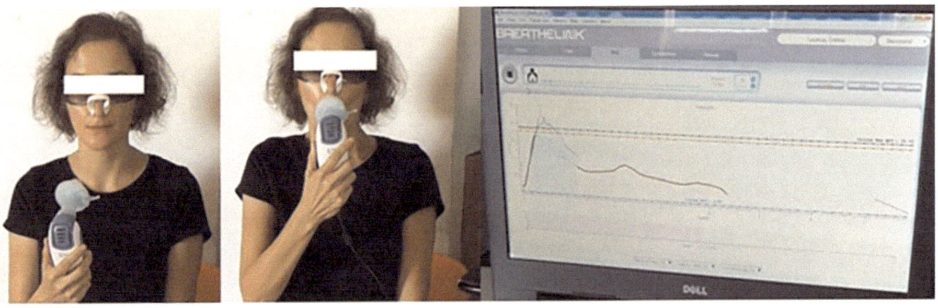

Figure 10.
Respiratory muscle pressure testing. Source photo: Respiratory Rehabilitation Clinic, Rehabilitation Clinical Hospital, Iasi, Romania, Head: Assoc. Prof. Dr. Paraschiva Postolache.

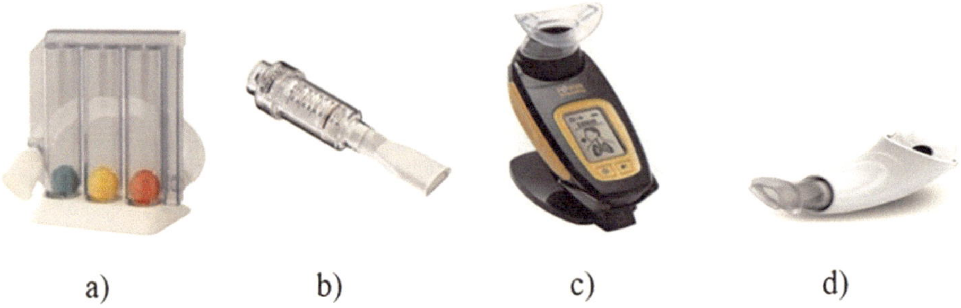

Figure 11.
Devices for training the respiratory muscles (a) stimulation spirometer; (b) Threshold; (c) POWERBreathe; and (d) Shaker Plus. Source photo: Respiratory Rehabilitation Clinic, Rehabilitation Clinical Hospital, Iasi, Romania, Head: Assoc. Prof. Dr. Paraschiva Postolache.

COPD patient (and not only) who remain symptomatic despite optimal therapy [39]. The purpose of respiratory muscle training is to improve respiratory muscle function, hypoxia, hypoventilation, and relieve dyspnea [40].

Before starting the training program, the maximum inspiratory pressure at the level of the oral cavity will be evaluated, which represents the exercise capacity of the inspiratory muscles, the methods and equipment used for the two types of training being significantly different (**Figure 10**) [41].

Respiratory muscle training involves training the inspiratory and expiratory muscles (**Figure 11**). Depending on the type of exercise, training can be strength (consisting of a series of repeated breaths with increased endurance) or endurance (forced ventilation maintained for several minutes). In general, inspiratory muscle training is used in patients with dyspnea, as a predominant symptom, and expiratory muscle training in patients with productive cough [42].

Respiratory muscle training should be continued after the discharge of patients from PR centers, daily, independently or in association with the PR program, at home, and, if possible, in specialized PR centers, at least two to three times a week, in order to maintain the effects of training [5].

5. Factors that limit the capacity of effort

The function of the respiratory and cardiovascular systems is adequately tested only during physical exertion. Each of the two systems has a reserve capacity well above that required to support the normal functioning of the body at rest and during moderate physical activity. Many pathologies that affect breathing or circulation cause progressive loss of physiological function. Such diseases are likely to be manifested initially by a reduction in lung or cardiac reserve. Because reserve abilities are tested only during exertion, the early (and potentially curable) stages of such diseases can only cause symptoms with exertion. By assessing the maximum capacity of patients to exercise, the pulmonologist or cardiologist assesses, at least in qualitative terms, the reserve capacity of each of the organ systems that contribute to the response to exertion [25].

Exercise performance reflects a coordinated response of respiratory and cardiovascular function along with the action of the muscles being trained. Physical exertion induces gradual increases in the frequency and depth of respiration, heart rate, blood pressure, heart rate, and myocardial contractility. During constant exertion, the respiratory and cardiovascular parameters begin to stabilize (after 1–2 minutes of rapid change) at appropriate levels, for a certain intensity of exercise in a certain patient. These balance levels can be used to characterize patient performance.

Effort capacity is the maximum amount of physical exertion a patient can endure, and exercise intolerance is a condition in which the patient is unable to exercise at the level and/or duration that would be expected from someone of his age and general physical condition (**Figure 12**).

Exercise intolerance in patients with chronic lung disease is multifactorial in nature, involving the following:

- *ventilatory abnormalities:*
    - during exercise of progressively increasing intensity, healthy elderly people can increase their breathing rate and current volume to provide an increase of up to 10–15 times the ventilation per minute, which is essential to eliminate the production of carbon dioxide and satisfies the increased oxygen demand → in such cases, ventilatory function is often not the limiting factor, at least for a wide range of submaximal stress levels, as ventilation per minute is maintained well below maximum ventilatory capacity (**Figure 13**);

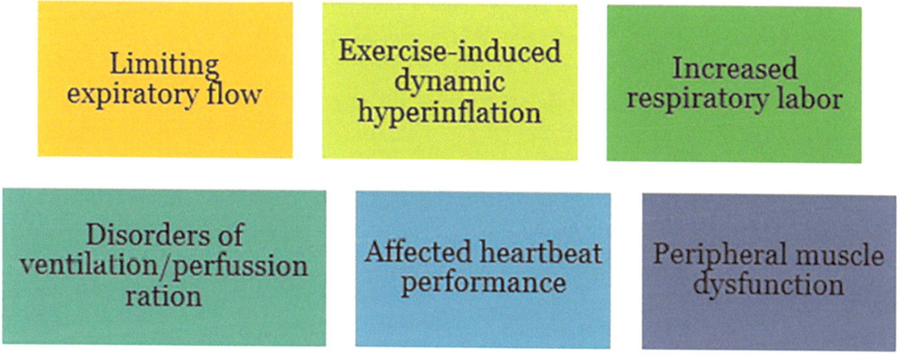

Figure 12.
Mechanisms that limit exercise capacity in chronic respiratory disease [7].

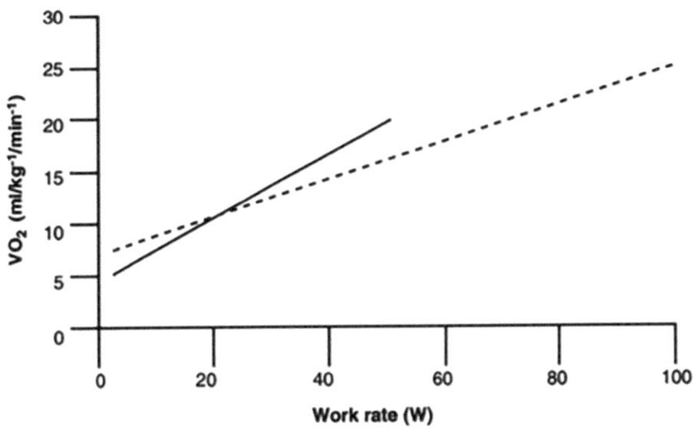

Figure 13.
Changing the oxygen consumption in relation to the working rate on a cycle ergometer, in a healthy person (dotted line), and in a patient with COPD (continuous line) [43].

- reduced ventilatory capacity during exercise is due to abnormal respiratory mechanics and respiratory muscle dysfunction;

- in patients with chronic respiratory disease, high resistance of the inspiratory and expiratory airways and/or reduced compliance may substantially increase the pressure required for airflow and thus my increase respiratory labor → the respiratory muscles are frequently weakened and unable to withstand adequately due to the presence of hyperinflation and/or intrinsic muscle dysfunction/hypoperfusion;

- a ventilatory demand is increased during physical exertion due to gas exchange abnormalities (e.g., change in ventilation/perfusion ratio and increased dead spate ventilation), which leads to hypoxemia and [28, 44–46].

- *gas exchange anomalies:*

    - despite the deterioration of the ventilatory reserve with aging, healthy elderly people seem to be able to maintain alveolar ventilation at a level that allows blood gases to be kept within normal limits, even during intense exercise → the ventilation/infusion ratio remains good because both ventilation, and the infusion increase several times with increasing exercise intensity → alveolo-capillary diffusion remains intact and, consequently, PaO_2 remains normal, even at high exercise intensities;

    - gas exchange regulation is affected in chronic lung disease producing various abnormalities of ventilation/perfusion ratio, diffusion disorders, and hypoxemia at rest and during exertion → many patients with severe lung disease experience arterial oxygen desaturation during exertion [28, 47–49].

- *cardiovascular disorders:*

    - cardiac output in healthy subjects may increase several times in response to physical exertion;

   - in chronic lung diseases, mechanisms involving oxygen transport are frequently affected, leading to a reduction in cardiovascular function:
   - first, coexisting right and left ventricular dysfunction can affect exercise capacity due to decreased cardiac output, which often leads to impaired oxygen delivery and early development of metabolic acidosis;
   - secondly, in chronic lung diseases, especially in the presence of pulmonary vascular abnormalities, pulmonary hypertension and right ventricular dysfunction may develop;
   - these phenomena may worsen in the presence of hyponemia → increased pulmonary vascular resistance and pulmonary arterial hypertension, with consecutive right heart failure;
   - increased cardiac output, along with low oxygen content, reduces systemic oxygen delivery to all organs of the body, including skeletal muscle [28, 50–53].

- *peripheral muscle dysfunction:*
   - inactivity, muscle deconditioning, and fatigue are associated with lower muscle mass and impaired muscle fiber distribution, especially with regard to the proportion of type I fibers (slow shrinking oxidative);
   - reducing the proportion of oxidative fibers reduces the oxidative potential of muscles, which are more prone to fatigue during high-intensity exercise;
   - structural and metabolic abnormalities of the limb muscles can lead to early lactic acidosis and failure of pregnancy due to exertion [54–57].

6. Conclusions

Patients with chronic lung disease have varying degrees of activity limitation due to skeletal and respiratory muscle dysfunction, a limitation that is remedied by physical training in the complex PR program.

Pulmonary rehabilitation is on the basic therapies, with strong scientific evidence and an essential role in the management of chronic respiratory diseases. PR is a valuable treatment tool, a source of measurement and information tools for respiratory pathophysiology.

As an essential part of chronic lung disease management, PR relieves dyspnea and fatigue, anxiety, and depression, improves exercise tolerance and health-related quality of life, and reduces the number of hospitalizations for exacerbations and mortality of patients with chronic lung disease. Exercise training is the key component of PR, which consists of exercise evaluation and actual training therapy. Exercise assessments are an important component of PR and should take into account patients' symptoms, endurance, strength, and health-related quality of life.

Dyspnea is an important symptom of chronic, multifaceted lung disease, and its understanding can be derived from a multidisciplinary and multidimensional approach.

The ability to walk is a quick and inexpressive measure of functional status and an important component of quality of life, reflecting a person's autonomy, which is significantly reduced in patients with chronic lung disease.

Functional measures at rest do not always provide an accurate diagnosis and adequate stratification of severity in patients with chronic respiratory disease. That is why cardiopulmonary exercise testing is necessary, which provides useful information about exercise capacity and a comprehensive assessment of pathological mechanisms that limit exercise tolerance.

Both respiratory and cardiovascular fitness and exercise capacity are key elements in pulmonary rehabilitation programs. These parameters allow for the optimal prescribing of exercise programs and the inclusion of patient in physical training groups, which will lead to an increase in the effectiveness and safety of lung rehabilitation therapy for chronic respiratory patients.

Conflict of interest

The authors declare no conflict of interest.

Author details

Paraschiva Postolache[1,2], Ștefan Săndulache[3]*, Constantin Ghimuș[3] and Alexandru Nechifor[4]

1 Respiratory Rehabilitation Clinic, Rehabilitation Clinical Hospital, Iasi, Romania

2 Department of Medical Specialties (I), "Grigore T. Popa" University of Medicine and Pharmacy, Iasi, Romania

3 Clinic of Pneumology, Clinical Hospital of Pneumophtisiology, Iasi, Romania

4 Department of Clinical Medicine, "Dunarea de Jos" University of Galati, Galați, Romania

*Address all correspondence to: stefan.sandulache94@yahoo.com

References

[1] Holland AE, Cox N, Houchen-Wolloff L, et al. Defining modern pulmonary rehabilitation an official American Thoracic Society workshop report. Annals of the American Thoracic Society. 2021;**18**(5):e12-e29. DOI: 10.1513/AnnalsATS.202102-146ST

[2] Spruit MA, Wouters FM. Organizational aspects of pulmonary rehabilitation in chronic respiratory diseases. Respirology. 2019;**24**:838-843. DOI: 10.1111/resp.13512

[3] Nici L, Donner C, Wouters E, et al. American Thoracic Society/European Respiratory Society statement on pulmonary rehabilitation. American Journal of Respiratory and Critical Care Medicine. 2006;**173**(12): 1390-1413. DOI: 10.1164/rccm.200508-1211ST

[4] Spruit MA, Singh SJ, Garvey C, et al. An official American Thoracic Society/ European Respiratory Society statement: Key concepts and advances in pulmonary rehabilitation. American Journal of Respiratory and Critical Care Medicine. 2013;**188**(8):e13-e64. DOI: 10.1164/rccm.201309-1634ST

[5] Rochester C, Vogiatzis I, Holland AE, et al. An official American Thoracic Society/European Respiratory Society policy statement: Enhancing implementation, use, and delivery of pulmonary rehabilitation. American Journal of Respiratory and Critical Care Medicine. 2015;**192**(11): 1373-1386. DOI: 10.1164/rccm.201510-1966ST

[6] Postolache AP, Marciniuk DD. Handbook of Pulmonary Rehabilitation. New York: Nova Science Publishers, Inc; 2021

[7] Donner C, Ambronsino N, Goldstein R. Pulmonary Rehabilitation. New York: CRC Press; 2021

[8] Rochester C, Spruit M, Holland A. Pulmonary rehabilitation in 2021. Journal of the American Medical Association. 2021;**326**(10):969-970. DOI: 10.1001/jama.2021.6560

[9] Postolache P, Săndulache Ș, Ghimuș C. Reabilitarea respiratorie în era COVID-19 și experiența unei clinici de referință din România. In: Voicu V coordonator, editor. Sechele post-COVID-19 sau boala post-COVID-19 prelungită (sindromul post-COVID-19). București: Editura Academiei Române; 2022. pp. 163-194

[10] Heatherton TF, Kozlowski LT, Frecker RC, Fagerström KO. The Fagerström test for nicotine dependence: A revision of the Fagerström tolerance questionnaire. British Journal of Addiction. 1991;**86**: 1119-1127. DOI: 10.1111/j.1360-0443.1991.tb01879.x

[11] Michielsen HJ, De Vries J, Van Heck GL. Psychometric qualities of a brief self-rated fatigue measure the fatigue assessment scale. Journal of Psychosomatic Research. 2003;**54**: 345-352. DOI: 10.1016/s0022-3999(02)00392-6

[12] Lawton MP, Brody EM. Assessment of older people: Self-maintaining and instrumental activities of daily living. The Gerontologist. 1969;**9**(3): 179-186

[13] Antinouri A, Arendt G, Becker JT, et al. Updated research nosology for HIV-associated neurocognitive disorders. Neurology. 2007;**69**(18):

1789-1799. DOI: 10.1212/01.WNL.0000287431.88658.8b

[14] Lins L, Martins CF. SF-36 total score as a single measure of health-related quality of life: Scoping review. SAGE Open Medical. 2016;**4**: 2050312116671725. DOI: 10.1177/2050312116671725

[15] Postolache PA. Romana LINQ Questionnaire. Lung Information Needs Questionnaire (LINQ). Available from: http://www.linq.org.uk/PDFquestionnaires/LINQRomana.pdf [Accesed: May 25, 2022]

[16] Croitoru A, Postolache P. Evaluation of COPD patients for the pulmonary rehabilitation. In: Postolache AP, Marciniuk DD, editors. Handbook of Pulmonary Rehabilitation. New York: Nova Science Publishers, Inc; 2021. pp. 41-64

[17] Postolache PA, Cojocaru DC. Pulmonary rehabilitation - from guidelines to practice. Revista Medico-Chirurgicală a Societății de Medici şi Naturalişti din Iaşi. 2013;**117**(2):380-387

[18] Sami R, Saleni K, Hashemi M, et al. Exploring the barriers to pulmonary rehabilitation for patients with chronic obstructive pulmonary disease: A qualitative study. BMC Health Services Research. 2021;**21**:828-834. DOI: 10.1186/s12913-021-06814-5

[19] Parshall M, Schwartzstein R, Adams L, et al. An official American Thoracic Society statement: Update on the mechanisms, assessment, and Management of Dyspnea. American Journal of Respiratory and Critical Care Medicine. 2012;**185**(4):435-452. DOI: 10.1164/rccm.201111-2042ST

[20] Bestall JC, Paul EA, Garrod R, et al. Usefulness of the Medical Research Council (MRC) dyspnoea scale as a measure of disability in patients with chronic obstructive pulmonary disease. Thorax. 1999;**54**(7):581-586. DOI: 10.1136/thx.54.7.581

[21] Mador MJ, Rodis A, Magalang UJ. Reproducibility of Borg scale measurements of dyspnea during exercise in patients with COPD. Chest. 1995;**107**(6):1590-1597. DOI: 10.1378/chest.107.6.1590

[22] Bausewein C, Farquhar M, Booth S, et al. Measurement of breathlessness in advanced disease: A systematic review. Respiratory Medicine. 2007;**101**(3): 399-410. DOI: 10.1016/j.rmed.2006.07.003

[23] Ren L, Li QY. Evaluation of pulmonary rehabilitation and BODE index. Chinese Journal of Rehabilitation Medicine. 2009;**2009**(08):763-765

[24] Stringer W, Marciniuk D. The role of cardiopulmonary exercise testing (CPET) in pulmonary rehabilitation (PR) of chronic obstructive pulmonary disease (COPD) patients. COPD. 2018; **15**(6):621-631. DOI: 10.1080/15412555.2018.1550476

[25] Chen L, Su J. Pulmonary rehabilitation exercise assessments and training methods for patients with COPD: A literature review. Journal of Rehabilitation Therapy. 2021;**3**(1):13-20

[26] Zeng Y, Jiang F, Chen Y, et al. Exercise assessments and trainings of pulmonary rehabilitation in COPD: A literature review. International Journal of Chronic Obstructive Pulmonary Disease. 2018;**13**:2013-2023. DOI: 10.2147/COPD.S167098

[27] Clini E, Holland E, Pitta F, Troosters T. Textbook of Pulmonary

Rehabilitation. Switzerland: Springer International Publishing AG; 2018

[28] Wasserman K. Exercise testing and interpretation: An overview. In: Weinberg WR, editor. Principles of Exercise Testing and Interpretation. Baltimore: Lippincott Williams & Wilkins; 2005. pp. 1-9

[29] American Thoracic Society, American College of Chest Physicians. ATS/ACCP statement on cardiopulmonary exercise testing. American Journal of Respiratory and Critical Care Medicine. 2003; **167**(2):211-277. DOI: 10.1164/rccm.167.2.211

[30] ERS Task Force, Palange P, Ward S, et al. Recommendations on the use of exercise testing in clinical practice. The European Respiratory Journal. 2007; **29**(1):185-209. DOI: 10.1183/09031936.00046906

[31] ATS Committee on proficiency standards for clinical pulmonary function laboratories. ATS statement: Guidelines for the six-minute walk test. American Journal of Respiratory and Critical Care Medicine. 2002;**166**(1): 111-117. DOI: 10.1164/ajrccm.166.1.at1102

[32] Jenkins S, Cecins N, Camarri B, et al. Regression equations to predict 6-minute walk distance in middle-aged and elderly adults. Physiotherapy Theory and Practice. 2009;**25**(7):516-522. DOI: 10.3109/09593980802664711

[33] Holland AE, Spruit MA, Troosters T, et al. An official European Respiratory Society/American Thoracic Society technical standard: Field walking tests in chronic respiratory disease. The European Respiratory Journal. 2014;**44**(6):1428-1446. DOI: 10.1183/09031936.00150314

[34] Fell B, Hanekom S, Heine M. Six-minute walk test protocol variations in low-resource settings – A scoping review. South African Journal of Physiotheraphy. 2021;**77**(1):1549

[35] Postolache P, Meca AD. Exercise program and prescription in pulmonary rehabilitation. In: Postolache AP, Marciniuk DD, editors. Handbook of Pulmonary Rehabilitation. New York: Nova Science Publishers, Inc; 2021. pp. 141-162

[36] Gloeck R, Schneeberger T, Jarosch I, et al. Pulmonary rehabilitation and exercise training in chronic obstructive pulmonary disease. Deutsches Ärzteblatt International. 2018;**115**(8):117-123. DOI: 10.3238/arztebl.2018.0117

[37] Chen H, Li P, Li N, et al. Rehabilitation effects of land and water-based aerobic exercise on lung function, dyspnea, and exercise capacity in patients with chronic obstructive pulmonary disease. Medicine (Baltimore). 2021;**100**(33):e26976. DOI: 10.1097/MD.0000000000026976

[38] Gloeckl R, Marinov B, Pitta F. Practical recommendations for exercise training in patients with COPD. European Respiratory Review. 2013;**22**: 178-186. DOI: 10.1183/09059180.00000513

[39] Postolache PA, Jimborean G, Ianoși ES, et al. Respiratory muscle training in chronic obstructive pulmonary disease. Pneumologia. 2017; **66**(3):128-131

[40] Hollebeke M, Gosselink R, Langer D. Training specificity of inspiratory muscle training methods: A randomized trial. Frontiers in Physiology. 2020;**11**:1-13. DOI: 10.3389/fphys.2020.576595

[41] Gohl OC. Respiratory muscle training - practical aspects. In: Postolache AP, Marciniuk DD, editors. Handbook of Pulmonary Rehabilitation. New York: Nova Science Publishers, Inc; 2021. pp. 181-192

[42] Jimborean G, Ianoşi ES, Postolache AP. Respiratory rehabilitation and respiratory muscle training. In: Postolache AP, Marciniuk DD, editors. Handbook of Pulmonary Rehabilitation. New York: Nova Science Publishers, Inc; 2021. pp. 163-179

[43] Palange P, Ward SA, Carlsen KH, et al. Recommendation on the use of exercise testing in clinical practice. The European Respiratory Journal. 2007;**29**:185-209. DOI: 10.1183/09031936.00046906

[44] Johnson BD, Badr MS, Dempsey JA. Impact of the aging pulmonary system on the response to exercise. Clinics in Chest Medicine. 1994;**15**(2):229-246

[45] Johnson BD, Reddan WG, Seow KC, et al. Flow limitation and regulation of functional residual capacity during exercise in a physically active aging population. The American Review of Respiratory Disease. 1991;**143**(5 Pt 1): 960-967

[46] Dillard TA, Piantadosi S, Rajagopal KR. Prediction of ventilation at maximal exercise in chronic airflow obstruction. The American Review of Respiratory Disease. 1985;**132**:230-235

[47] O'Donnell DE. Exercise limitation and clinical exercise testing in chronic obstructive pulmonary disease. In: Weisman I, Zeballos R, editors. Progress in Respiratory Research. Basel: Karger; 2002. pp. 138-158

[48] Rice AJ, Thornton A, Gore C, et al. Pulmonary gas exchange during exercise in highly trained cyclists with arterial hypoxemia. Journal of Applied Physiology. 1999;**87**(5):1802-1812

[49] O'Donnell DE, Ofir D, Laveneziana P. Patterns of cardiopulmonary response to exercise in lung diseases. In: European Respiratory Monograph. United Kingdom: European Respiratory Society; 2007. pp. 69-92

[50] Naeije R. Pulmonary hypertension and right heart failure in chronic obstructive pulmonary disease. Proceedings of the American Thoracic Society. 2005;**2**(1):20-22. DOI: 10.1513/pats.200407-037MS

[51] Agusti AG, Barbera J, Roca J, et al. Hypoxic pulmonary vasoconstriction and gas exchange during exercise in chronic obstructive pulmonary disease. Chest. 1990;**97**(2):268-275. DOI: 10.1378/chest.97.2.268

[52] Dantzker DR, D'Alonzo GE. The effect of exercise in pulmonary gas exchange in patients with severe chronic obstructive pulmonary disease. The American Review of Respiratory Disease. 1986;**134**(6):1135-1139. DOI: 10.1164/arrd.1986.134.6.1135

[53] Prampero PE. Factors limiting maximal performance in humans. European Journal of Applied Physiology. 2003;**90**(3–4):420-429

[54] Gosselink R, Troosters T, Decramer M. Peripheral muscle weakness contributes to exercise limitation in COPD. American Journal of Respiratory Critical Care Medical Science and Sports Exercise. 1996; **153**(3):976-980. DOI: 10.1164/ajrccm.153.3.8630582

[55] Hamilton AL, Killian K, Summers E, et al. Muscle strength, symptom intensity, and exercise capacity in

patients with cardiorespiratory disorders. American Journal of Respiratory and Critical Care Medicine. 1995;**152**(6 Pt 1):2021-2031. DOI: 10.1164/ajrccm.152.6.8520771

[56] Serres I, Gautier V, Varray A, et al. Impaired skeletal muscle endurance related to physical inactivity and altered lung function in COPD patients. Chest. 1998;**113**(4):900-905. DOI: 10.1378/chest.113.4.900

[57] Farooqi MAM, Killian K, Satia I. The impact of muscle strength on exercise capacity and symptoms. ERJ Open Research. 2020;**6**:00089-02020. DOI: 10.1183/23120541.00089-2020

Chapter 3

Promoting Cardiorespiratory Fitness in Young People: The Importance of the School Context

Miguel Peralta, Sandra Martins, Duarte Henriques-Neto, Riki Tesler and Adilson Marques

Abstract

The ability to deliver oxygen to the skeletal muscles and use it to generate energy to support muscle activity is known as cardiorespiratory fitness (CRF). Because of its importance to health, young people's declining CRF is a cause of concern. Therefore, promoting CRF through physical activity (PA) participation is needed. Among young people, the school setting has been proposed as a privileged context to promote PA and CRF, and school-based PA interventions are known to improve PA and CRF. Nevertheless, school-based PA interventions are not universal and may not be sustainable over long periods if the mobilized resources are not sustained. There is a need to promote sustainable health promotion actions to maintain their benefits beyond the initial stage of implementation and deliver within the limits of the available resources. One way of doing so is through physical education (PE). PE is part of the curriculum in most countries, allows children and adolescents to engage in PA, and is supervised by trained PE teachers. The school is a privileged context for health promotion actions through its regular implementation across most education years. This chapter advocates PE as a privileged setting for promoting PA and CRF.

Keywords: adolescent, children, health, physical activity, physical education

1. Introduction

The terms physical activity (PA), exercise and physical fitness are often used interchangeably since they are closely related. However, they do not represent the same construct. This distinction is of importance as throughout the text, these terms will be used often. Thus, it is perhaps best to start by defining each one. PA can be defined as any body movement produced by the skeletal muscle that results in energy expenditure [1]. PA represents a full range of intensities, including light intensity PA (<3 metabolic equivalents of task), moderate-intensity PA (≥3 and < 6 metabolic equivalents of task) and vigorous-intensity PA (≥6 metabolic equivalents of task) [2]. On the other hand, exercise is a normally planned and structured subcategory of PA.

It requires repetitive body movements to maintain or improve one or more components of physical fitness [1]. Lastly, physical fitness is a multi-component construct that can be understood as a set of attributes an individual has or can achieve. From a broader perspective, physical fitness is a physiologic attribute representing an individual's capacity to perform muscle-powered activities [3]. Physical fitness can be divided into health-related and skill-related components. Health-related physical fitness includes cardiorespiratory fitness (CRF), muscular strength, muscular endurance, muscular flexibility, and body composition [1]. Independently of physical activity, health-related physical fitness is linked to a lower prevalence of chronic disease and has a strong relationship with health and wellness [3].

The most studied health-related component of physical fitness is the CRF. CRF relates to the capacity of the circulatory and respiratory systems to supply oxygen to muscles during a sustained physical effort, that is, reflects the capacity of the respiratory and cardiovascular systems to bear prolonged exercise [4]. Even though a large part of the variability of CRF, up to half, is biologically and genetically determined [5], hereditability is not the only determinant of CRF. Socio-environmental factors and PA, particularly exercise, also influence CRF to a large extent [6].

Childhood and adolescence are crucial periods of life marked by several morphological, physiological, psychological, and behavioural changes. Sex and maturity are two determinants of CRF that shape its improvement at these ages. It is widely known that boys' CRF is higher than girls', from late childhood onward. This difference increases throughout adolescence, reaching about a 40% gap in post-pubertal 18-year-old boys. This difference is greatly explained by boys' marked increase in fat-free mass (about 90% increase between 11 and 16 years old, compared to a 40% increase in girls) driven by maturation [7]. Besides sex, maturity status is also an important determinant of CRF, as the growth and development processes are not linear and do not happen simultaneously in young people, between and within each sex.

Although CRF is mostly dependent on genetics, sex, and maturation, other environmental and behavioural factors are also important for aerobic capacities, such as weight status, sleep, nutrition or PA levels. Among those factors, PA has the greatest impact on CRF. Engaging in PA and exercise activates almost all biological systems to support the muscle contraction and energy production [8]. In response to PA, the cardiovascular and respiratory systems increase oxygen availability for energy production in the muscle; when regularly stimulated, muscles improve their ability to function optimally. Therefore, PA is considered the primary means of promoting CRF [6]. Within PA, exercise seems to contribute the most to improvements in CRF, mainly because of the higher activity intensity and regularity of practice. Engaging in regular moderate-to-vigorous, especially vigorous, PA is most beneficial for improving CRF [9]. Also, previous investigations have demonstrated that children and adolescents participating in organised sports have better CRF than their non-participating peers and that appropriate exercise training is known to increase CRF levels in youth, irrespective of sex, age or maturity [10, 11]. More specifically, programmes to benefit CRF usually involve 20–45-minute sessions of continuous moderate-to-vigorous or vigorous-intensity training or high-intensity interval training over at least 2 to 3 months [10, 12].

PA, exercise and physical fitness are the related concepts that warrant differential interpretations. Furthermore, PA, especially higher intensity, exercise and CRF are positively associated. Because of that, better CRF performances can be seen as a marker of PA levels, total amount or volume essentially of higher intensities, with evidence highlighting vigorous activities. Therefore, from a monitoring perspective,

CRF provides a robust measure and stable reflection of recent and past PA levels and indicates biological system functioning [6].

2. Cardiorespiratory fitness and health

The health benefit evidence of PA and fitness, namely CRF, in children and adolescents is undisputable. For that reason, promoting PA and healthy lifestyles has become a priority for education and health authorities worldwide [13]. Among young people, engaging in PA and having better physical fitness are beneficial for several health outcomes, such as obesity, cardiometabolic health, bone health and mental health, as well as for pro-social behaviour, sleep, and cognitive outcomes [2]. Promoting PA has been consistently shown to be an effective strategy to improve health in general and is considered as a 'best buy' in health promotion [14].

In youth, regular PA is positively associated with beneficial cardiometabolic health outcomes, including improved blood pressure, lipid profile, glucose control, insulin sensitivity and bone health, while being inversely associated with overweight and obesity [2]. Furthermore, the benefits of PA seem to be greater with increasing intensity. For example, children and adolescents who engage in higher levels of PA have lower resting blood pressure and triglyceride concentration [15] and more favourable indicators of arterial stiffness [16]. Also, recent evidence reinforces the idea that PA, especially when participating in 30–60 minutes of moderate-to-vigorous PA for three or more days per week, improves CRF and musculoskeletal fitness in children and adolescents [3]. Besides physical health, the promotion of mental health and the development and maintenance of cognitive function are essential across the entire lifespan. Scientific evidence has shown that PA has positive effects on overall mental health and health-related quality of life [3, 17], and the prevention or treatment of depression and anxiety [18]. Furthermore, PA has positive effects on cognitive function and academic outcomes [19, 20].

Several hypotheses have been proposed regarding the underlying mechanisms responsible for the effects of PA on mental health. On a physiological level, PA may promote mental health by releasing endorphins and neurogenesis [21, 22]. On a psychological level, PA is associated with several aspects related to mental health, such as positive relationships with others, social learning, making new friends and self-esteem [22, 23].

Independently of PA, CRF is a well-known indicator of young peoples' current and future health [24], which is associated with cardiovascular health, cholesterol and blood lipids levels, obesity and mental health [25, 26]. **Figure 1** summarises the associations between CRF and health in youth.

Children and adolescents with greater CRF levels have healthier cardiovascular and metabolic profiles [25]. Furthermore, CRF is inversely associated with total adiposity, and having high levels of CRF can counteract the harmful consequences attributed to having a higher inflammatory profile [25, 26]. Therefore, CRF is related to the clustering of cardiometabolic risk factors and is an important marker of health [27]. CRF is also associated with mental health in youth. CRF is related to greater global grey and white matter, brain volume and anterior hippocampal functional connectivity [28]. This is of importance and may explain why, among adolescents, higher CRF is related to better academic performance [20].

Although the adverse effects of non-communicable diseases are mainly manifested in adults and older adults, it is evident that the development of these conditions

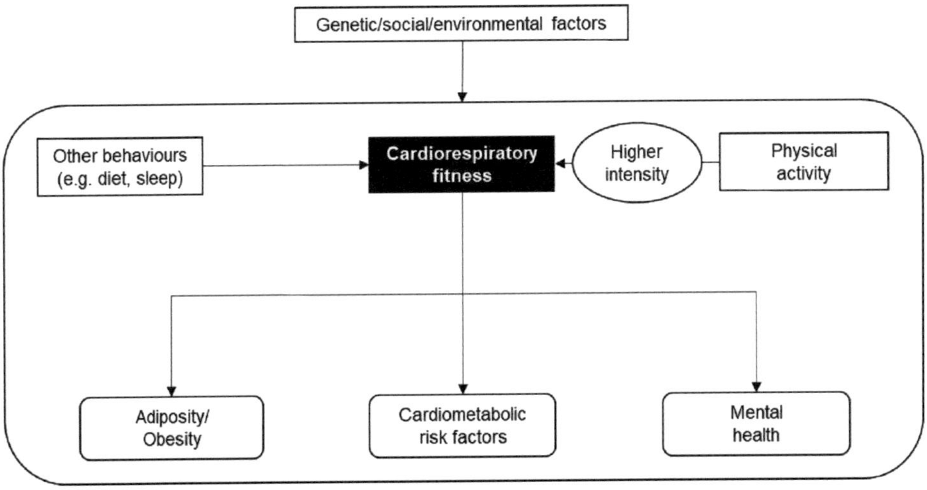

Figure 1.
Associations between cardiorespiratory fitness and several health outcomes in children and adolescents (adapted from [25]).

may start much earlier in life. Additionally, it is known that CRF moderately tracks from childhood to adolescence and from adolescence to adulthood [29]. Therefore, it seems reasonable to conclude that promoting PA and physical fitness, including CRF, in young people is essential to nurture healthy lifestyles that may help to prevent present and future non-communicable diseases and take the right steps to a healthier population.

PA is an important health behaviour [2], and CRF is a powerful marker of health [25], so PA should be part of our daily routine. Considering this evidence, the World Health Organization (WHO) recommends children and adolescents aged 5–17 years old engage in at least 60 minutes of daily moderate-to-vigorous PA to achieve the health benefits [2]. It is further recommended that most of the daily PA be aerobic and that muscle-strengthening activities should be performed at least three times per week [2]. Also, considering the health benefit of greater CRF, several specialists have stressed the importance of improving and promoting CRF in children and adolescents [6, 25, 26].

3. What are the current cardiorespiratory fitness levels?

Despite the health benefits summarised previously, PA and CRF levels among young people are low and declining globally. Using a pooled analysis of cross-sectional survey data from 146 countries, recent evidence suggests that 81% of children and adolescents aged 11–17 do not meet the current recommendations for daily PA [30]. It was further observed that more girls than boys were insufficiently active in 2016, respectively 84.7% and 77.6%. Similarly, the global matrix 3.0 PA report card project, which graded evidence to harmonise available data from 49 countries worldwide, has suggested that children and adolescents have low compliance with the WHO PA guidelines, and only 27–33% (grade D) met the PA recommendations [31].

In adults, insufficient PA has been identified as one of the leading risk factors for premature mortality and disease burden [32]. Thus, the low PA levels in children and adolescents are alarming as they are associated with lower physical activity levels later in life [33] and might be one of the causes for the declining trend observed in CRF worldwide in this population [34]. In a trend analysis from 1981 to 2014, Tomkinson et al. [34] verified a moderate decline in young people's CRF living in 19 high-income and upper-middle-income countries between these years (−7.3% change). Furthermore, a substantial decline since 1981 was observed, which has slowed and stabilised internationally since 2000.

Given the health benefits of being physically active and fit worldwide, there is a concerning declining trend in both PA and CRF. Exactly because of that, the WHO has declared that one of their global health initiatives is to increase the populations' PA levels and reduce by 10% the prevalence of insufficient PA by 2025 [35]. Therefore, there is an imperative need to develop strategies for the promotion of PA and CRF at the population level that are effective and sustainable.

4. The role of school in promoting cardiorespiratory fitness

Promoting PA and healthy lifestyles has become a priority for public health authorities worldwide [13]. There are several contexts to consider when developing PA and fitness promotion strategies among children and adolescents, including organised sports participation, active commuting, unstructured leisure time and school [13, 36].

School is considered an important setting for health promotion among children and adolescents, and PA and CRF are no exception [36]. It is recognised that the single most important channel to address physical inactivity in youth is through school [35, 37]. Comprehensive whole-of-school approaches represent an effective strategy to address young people's physical inactivity levels [38]. The role of the school extends to encouraging children and adolescents to continue engaging in PA by providing coordinated opportunities for all young people and developing partnerships with the wider community, in the both health and sports sectors, to extend and improve the opportunities available for students to remain physically active [39].

Several reasons contribute to the proclamation of schools as a priority setting for promoting PA and fitness. In the first place, schools provide opportunities for children and adolescents to engage in PA during discrete periods of the day, including PE, recess, school sports programmes and other extra-curricular programmes. This is especially important when considering youth from disadvantaged settings who have less access to PA [40]. Secondly, many children and adolescents spend a great part of the day at school. School-based interventions are the most universally applicable and effective way to counteract low PA and fitness since children and adolescents spend at least half of their waking hours in this setting [39]. Lastly, school is mandatory for children and adolescents in most countries worldwide. Thus, its programmes reach many young people [40].

There is considerable evidence from middle- and high-income countries that school-based health interventions moderately promote PA and CRF [41]. Thus, from a health promotion perspective, the school has been proposed as an important setting to promote PA and CRF. However, there is a gap between demonstrating the effectiveness of such PA interventions and understanding the wide-scale implementation and/or dissemination of these interventions [39]. Furthermore, these interventions are not universal and may not be sustainable over long periods if senior leaders and staff that are knowledgeable, skilled and motivated to continue delivering health promotion through ever-changing circumstances are not retained [42]. The implementation of effective school-based models into the real world setting is complex. It demands a multi-partner investment over the long term. Ecological approaches that integrate existing resources and institutions in the community are likely key to successful and sustained implementation [39]. Therefore, there is a need to promote sustainable health promotion actions that can maintain their benefits for communities and populations beyond their initial implementation stage and deliver within the limits of finances. One possibility for such action is through PE, which is already within the scope and budget of schools.

5. Physical education as an important setting to promote cardiorespiratory fitness

The importance of PE to promote health is widely recognised, as PE is by far the most common method of promoting PA during the school day [40]. PE, part of the school curriculum in most countries, allows children and adolescents to engage in structured, specialist-led, and appropriate PA. Particularly through PE, the school provides an opportunity for youth to be physically active and promote healthy lifestyles. In line with promoting health-enhancing PA, schools and PE are also important for promoting physical fitness. When performed appropriately and incorporated as one component of a broad and holistic health education programme, fitness monitoring in PE is a valuable part of the curriculum. It supports healthy lifestyles and PA [43].

One of the reasons why PE comprises a primacy setting for health promotion is throughout formative development, which can influence positive attitudes and behaviours of young people during compulsory school attendance years [39]. PE makes a unique contribution to health education through the development of physical and health literacy, where students are prompt to develop the necessary skills to make healthy choices, but also through providing opportunities to engage in PA and promote fitness [37, 39]. Additionally, PE is, for the most of school curricula worldwide, the subject focused on the body's movement and physical development, helping young people to learn, respect and value their bodies and abilities [39].

PE is the only setting where all children, especially those from low socio-economic status and girls, have access to moderate-to-vigorous PA and learn important fundamental movement skills that may provide the foundation for a lifetime of PA [40, 43]. It has been shown that PE classes contribute to an increase in daily moderate-to-vigorous PA in children and adolescents [44, 45]. It is estimated that PE lessons increase daily moderate-to-vigorous PA in about 12.8 minutes compared to days without PE lessons [46]. Furthermore, PA opportunities in PE are often regular, mostly two to three times a week, and represent the most of school-based PA [47]. Participation in PE was determined as the single most important determinant of school-based PA recommendations of at least 500 steps per hour, at least 25% of school time spent in PA, and at least 20 minutes of moderate-to-vigorous PA [47]. This is especially important when considering the promotion of fitness as regular higher-intensity PA is critical for improving it [6]. Due to its importance PE guidelines often recommend that at least 50% of class time should be spent in moderate-to-vigorous PA [37, 48].

Another important aspect related to PA offered in PE is the structuring and appropriateness of PA delivered [43, 49]. PE is often delivered by specialists, namely

PE teachers, with adequate training and capable of providing meaningful PA [50]. It is known that PE delivered by well-trained specialists increases PA during school hours in youth [37]. Furthermore, promoting PA and fitness in PE captures more than just the intensity of PA provided during the classes. Young people are more likely to engage in activities both in-class and outside of school, when activities are perceived as inherently meaningful, interesting and enjoyable, or hold personal relevance. Thus, Haerens et al. [51] argue that PE can only promote an active lifestyle if the activities provided have these characteristics. This view is supported by the self-determination theory [52] and reinforces the importance of promoting intrinsic motivation in PE. In this sense, PE teachers also have an important role in encouraging PA and fitness, as well as providing positive feedback which is associated with greater intentions to participate in PA [53].

Besides the important action of PE in promoting PA and CRF in children and adolescents, it also has an important role in monitoring and informing about students' CRF. Therefore, PE teachers have several quality tools to assess the students' CRF. Several field tests allow CRF assessment in the school setting and whole school classes to be assessed in one session. The most commonly used field-based CRF tests in the school setting are the Progressive Aerobic Cardiovascular Endurance Run (PACER), also known as the beep test or the 20-meter shuttle run, the 1-mile test and the Cooper test. Notwithstanding, fitness testing in PE, including CRF tests, should be done within a positive and health-promoting context [54]. For that it is recommended that teachers: a) provide meaningful practice opportunities so students become familiar with and develop value toward the tests, b) work with students to create personal goals toward physical fitness, and c) track individual progress across time.

6. Conclusion

CRF can be defined as the ability of the body to deliver atmosphere oxygen to the skeletal muscles and use it to generate energy to support muscle activity during exercise. CRF is associated with present and future cardiometabolic health, an important health marker [24]. Although up to half of the CRF is hereditable, participation in PA has still been considered the primary means of improving fitness [6]. Despite its associations with health, recent evidence has shown a substantial decline in CRF since 1981 in upper-middle- and high-income countries [34], which is a cause of concern.

The school has been proposed as an important setting to promote PA and CRF. School-based PA interventions are the effective strategies to promote children's and adolescents' PA levels and CRF [36]. However, these interventions are not universal and may not be sustainable over long periods if senior leaders and staff that are knowledgeable, skilled and motivated to continue delivering health promotion through ever-changing circumstances are not retained [42]. Therefore, there is a need to promote sustainable health promotion actions that can maintain their benefits beyond the initial stage of implementation and deliver within the limits of the available resources.

Within the school activities, PE, which is part of the school curriculum in most countries, allows children and adolescents to engage in structured and appropriate PA [43]. Thus, school is a privileged context for health promotion actions through its regular implementation across most education years.

Author details

Miguel Peralta[1], Sandra Martins[2], Duarte Henriques-Neto[3], Riki Tesler[4] and Adilson Marques[1*]

1 Faculdade de Motricidade Humana, Universidade de Lisboa, Lisboa, Portugal

2 Escola de Ciências da Saúde, Universidade Europeia, Lisboa, Portugal

3 Research Center in Sports Sciences, Health Sciences and Human Development, Maia University, Maia, Portugal

4 School of Health Sciences, Ariel University, Ariel, Israel

*Address all correspondence to: adncmpt@gmail.com

References

[1] Caspersen C, Powell K, Christenson G. Physical activity, exercise, and physical fitness: Definitions and distinctions for health-related research. Public Health Reports. 1985;**100**:126-131

[2] Bull FC, Al-Ansari SS, Biddle S, Borodulin K, Buman MP, Cardon G, et al. World Health Organization 2020 guidelines on physical activity and sedentary behaviour. British Journal of Sports Medicine. 2020;**54**(24):1451-1462. DOI: 10.1136/bjsports-2020-102955

[3] USDHHS. 2018 Physical Activity Guidelines Advisory Committee Scientific Report. 2018

[4] Taylor HL, Buskirk E, Henschel A. Maximal oxygen intake as an objective measure of cardio-respiratory performance. Journal of Applied Physiology. 1955;**8**(1):73-80. DOI: 10.1152/jappl.1955.8.1.73

[5] Ross R, Goodpaster BH, Koch LG, Sarzynski MA, Kohrt WM, Johannsen NM, et al. Precision exercise medicine: Understanding exercise response variability. British Journal of Sports Medicine. 2019;**53**(18):1141-1153. DOI: 10.1136/bjsports-2018-100328

[6] Lang JJ, Tomkinson GR, Janssen I, Ruiz JR, Ortega FB, Leger L, et al. Making a case for cardiorespiratory fitness surveillance among children and youth. Exercise and Sport Sciences Reviews. 2018;**46**(2):66-75. DOI: 10.1249/JES.0000000000000138

[7] Armstrong N, Welsman J. Sex-specific longitudinal modeling of youth peak oxygen uptake. Pediatric Exercise Science. 2019;**31**(2):204-212. DOI: 10.1123/pes.2018-0175

[8] Bouchard C, Blair SN, Haskell W. Physical Activity and Health. 2nd ed. Human Kinetics; 2012 Available from: https://books.google.pt/books?id=BpKE8PpcPR4C

[9] Collings PJ, Westgate K, Vaisto J, Wijndaele K, Atkin AJ, Haapala EA, et al. Cross-sectional associations of objectively-measured physical activity and sedentary time with body composition and cardiorespiratory fitness in mid-childhood: The PANIC study. Sports Medicine. 2017;**47**(4):769-780. DOI: 10.1007/s40279-016-0606-x

[10] Armstrong N, Barker AR. Endurance training and elite young athletes. Medicine and Sport Science. 2011;**56**:59-83. DOI: 10.1159/000320633

[11] Silva G, Andersen LB, Aires L, Mota J, Oliveira J, Ribeiro JC. Associations between sports participation, levels of moderate to vigorous physical activity and cardiorespiratory fitness in childrenand adolescents. Journal of Sports Sciences. 2013;**31**(12):1359-1367. DOI: 10.1080/02640414.2013.781666

[12] Baquet G, Berthoin S, Dupont G, Blondel N, Fabre C, van Praagh E. Effects of high intensity intermittent training on peak VO(2) in prepubertal children. International Journal of Sports Medicine. 2002;**23**(6):439-444. DOI: 10.1055/s-2002-33742

[13] WHO. Global Action Plan on Physical Activity 2018-2030: More Active People for a Healthier World. 2018

[14] WHO. Tackling NCDs: 'Best Buys' and Other Recommended Interventions for the Prevention and Control of Noncommunicable Diseases. Geneva, Switzerland: World Health Organization; 2017

[15] Cesa CC, Sbruzzi G, Ribeiro RA, Barbiero SM, de Oliveira Petkowicz R, Eibel B, et al. Physical activity and cardiovascular risk factors in children: meta-analysis of randomized clinical trials. Preventive Medicine. 2014;**69**:54-62. DOI: 10.1016/j.ypmed.2014.08.014

[16] Heil L, Oberhoffer R, Bohm B. Association between physical activity intensity levels and arterial stiffness in healthy children. Journal of Physical Activity and Health. 2020;**17**(10):933-939. DOI: 10.1123/jpah.2019-0594

[17] Biddle SJ, Asare M. Physical activity and mental health in children and adolescents: A review of reviews. British Journal of Sports Medicine. 2011;**45**(11):886-895. DOI: 10.1136/bjsports-2011-090185

[18] Korczak DJ, Madigan S, Colasanto M. Children's physical activity and depression: A Meta-analysis. Pediatrics. 2017;**139**(4):e20162266. DOI: 10.1542/peds.2016-2266

[19] Alvarez-Bueno C, Pesce C, Cavero-Redondo I, Sanchez-Lopez M, Martinez-Hortelano JA, Martinez-Vizcaino V. The effect of physical activity interventions on Children's cognition and metacognition: A systematic review and Meta-analysis. Journal of the American Academy of Child and Adolescent Psychiatry. 2017;**56**(9):729-738. DOI: 10.1016/j.jaac.2017.06.012

[20] Marques A, Santos DA, Hillman CH, Sardinha LB. How does academic achievement relate to cardiorespiratory fitness, self-reported physical activity and objectively reported physical activity: A systematic review in children and adolescents aged 6-18 years. British Journal of Sports Medicine. 2018;**52**(16):1039-1039. DOI: 10.1136/bjsports-2016-097361

[21] Cotman CW, Berchtold NC, Christie LA. Exercise builds brain health: Key roles of growth factor cascades and inflammation. Trends in Neurosciences. 2007;**30**(9):464-472. DOI: 10.1016/j.tins.2007.06.011

[22] Lubans D, Richards J, Hillman C, Faulkner G, Beauchamp M, Nilsson M, et al. Physical activity for cognitive and mental health in youth: A systematic review of mechanisms. Pediatrics. 2016;**138**(3):e20161642. DOI: 10.1542/peds.2016-1642

[23] Eime RM, Young JA, Harvey JT, Charity MJ, Payne WR. A systematic review of the psychological and social benefits of participation in sport for children and adolescents: Informing development of a conceptual model of health through sport. International Journal of Behavioral Nutrition and Physical Activity. 2013;**10**:98. DOI: 10.1186/1479-5868-10-98

[24] Henriksson P, Shiroma EJ, Henriksson H, Tynelius P, Berglind D, Lof M, et al. Fit for life? Low cardiorespiratory fitness in adolescence is associated with a higher burden of future disability. British Journal of Sports Medicine. 2021;**55**(3):128-129. DOI: 10.1136/bjsports-2020-102605

[25] Ortega FB, Ruiz JR, Castillo MJ, Sjostrom M. Physical fitness in childhood and adolescence: A powerful marker of health. International Journal of Obesity. 2008;**32**(1):1-11. DOI: 10.1038/sj.ijo.0803774

[26] Ruiz JR, Castro-Pinero J, Artero EG, Ortega FB, Sjostrom M, Suni J, et al. Predictive validity of health-related fitness in youth: A systematic review. British Journal of Sports Medicine. 2009;**43**(12):909-923. DOI: 10.1136/bjsm.2008.056499

[27] Anderssen SA, Cooper AR, Riddoch C, Sardinha LB, Harro M, Brage S, et al. Low cardiorespiratory fitness is a strong predictor for clustering of cardiovascular disease risk factors in children independent of country, age and sex. European Journal of Cardiovascular Prevention and Rehabilitation. 2007;**14**(4):526-531. DOI: 10.1097/HJR.0b013e328011efc1

[28] Esteban-Cornejo I, Stillman CM, Rodriguez-Ayllon M, Kramer AF, Hillman CH, Catena A, et al. Physical fitness, hippocampal functional connectivity and academic performance in children with overweight/obesity: The ActiveBrains project. Brain, Behavior, and Immunity. 2021;**91**:284-295. DOI: 10.1016/j.bbi.2020.10.006

[29] Twisk JW, Kemper HC, van Mechelen W. Tracking of activity and fitness and the relationship with cardiovascular disease risk factors. Medicine and Science in Sports and Exercise. 2000;**32**(8):1455-1461. DOI:10.1097/00005768-200008000-00014

[30] Guthold R, Stevens GA, Riley LM, Bull FC. Global trends in insufficient physical activity among adolescents: A pooled analysis of 298 population-based surveys with 1.6 million participants. Lancet Child Adolesc Health. 2020;**4**(1):23-35. DOI: 10.1016/S2352-4642(19)30323-2

[31] Aubert S, Barnes JD, Abdeta C, Abi Nader P, Adeniyi AF, Aguilar-Farias N, et al. Global matrix 3.0 physical activity report card grades for children and youth: Results and analysis from 49 countries. Journal of Physical Activity & Health. 2018;**15**(S2):S251-S273. DOI: 10.1123/jpah.2018-0472

[32] Ding D, Lawson KD, Kolbe-Alexander TL, Finkelstein EA, Katzmarzyk PT, van Mechelen W, et al. The economic burden of physical inactivity: A global analysis of major non-communicable diseases. Lancet. 2016;**388**(10051):1311-1324. DOI: 10.1016/S0140-6736(16)30383-X

[33] Telama R, Yang X, Leskinen E, Kankaanpaa A, Hirvensalo M, Tammelin T, et al. Tracking of physical activity from early childhood through youth into adulthood [research support, non-U.S. Gov't]. Medicine and Science in Sports and Exercise. 2014;**46**(5):955-962. DOI: 10.1249/MSS.0000000000000181

[34] Tomkinson GR, Lang JJ, Tremblay MS. Temporal trends in the cardiorespiratory fitness of children and adolescents representing 19 high-income and upper middle-income countries between 1981 and 2014. British Journal of Sports Medicine. 2019;**53**(8):478-486. DOI: 10.1136/bjsports-2017-097982

[35] WHO Regional Office for Europe. Physical Activity Strategy for the WHO European Region 2016-2025. Copenhagen: World Health Organization; 2016

[36] Messing S, Rutten A, Abu-Omar K, Ungerer-Rohrich U, Goodwin L, Burlacu I, et al. How can physical activity Be promoted among children and adolescents? A systematic review of reviews across settings. Frontiers in Public Health. 2019;7:55. DOI: 10.3389/fpubh.2019.00055

[37] IOM. The effectiveness of physical activity and physical education policies and programs: Summary of the evidence. In: Kohl HW III, Cook HD, editors. Educating the Student Body: Taking Physical Activity and Physical Education to School. The National Academies Press; 2013. pp. 311-364

[38] Naylor PJ, McKay HA. Prevention in the first place: Schools a setting for action

on physical inactivity. British Journal of Sports Medicine. 2009;**43**(1):10-13. DOI: 10.1136/bjsm.2008.053447

[39] Mountjoy M, Andersen LB, Armstrong N, Biddle S, Boreham C, Bedenbeck HP, et al. International Olympic Committee consensus statement on the health and fitness of young people through physical activity and sport. British Journal of Sports Medicine. 2011;**45**(11):839-848. DOI: 10.1136/bjsports-2011-090228

[40] Hills AP, Dengel DR, Lubans DR. Supporting public health priorities: Recommendations for physical education and physical activity promotion in schools. Progress in Cardiovascular Diseases. 2015;**57**(4):368-374. DOI: 10.1016/j.pcad.2014.09.010

[41] Hartwig TB, Sanders T, Vasconcellos D, Noetel M, Parker PD, Lubans DR, et al. School-based interventions modestly increase physical activity and cardiorespiratory fitness but are least effective for youth who need them most: An individual participant pooled analysis of 20 controlled trials. British Journal of Sports Medicine. 2021;**55**(13):721-729. DOI: 10.1136/bjsports-2020-102740

[42] Herlitz L, MacIntyre H, Osborn T, Bonell C. The sustainability of public health interventions in schools: A systematic review. Implementation Science. 2020;**15**(1):4. DOI: 10.1186/s13012-019-0961-8

[43] Harris J, Cale L. Promoting Active Lifestyles in Schools. Human Kinetics; 2019

[44] Froberg A, Raustorp A, Pagels P, Larsson C, Boldemann C. Levels of physical activity during physical education lessons in Sweden. Acta Paediatrica. 2017;**106**(1):135-141. DOI: 10.1111/apa.13551

[45] Hollis JL, Sutherland R, Williams AJ, Campbell E, Nathan N, Wolfenden L, et al. A systematic review and meta-analysis of moderate-to-vigorous physical activity levels in secondary school physical education lessons. International Journal of Behavioral Nutrition and Physical Activity. 2017;**14**(1):52. DOI: 10.1186/s12966-017-0504-0

[46] Mooses K, Pihu M, Riso EM, Hannus A, Kaasik P, Kull M. Physical education increases daily moderate to vigorous physical activity and reduces sedentary time. Journal of School Health. 2017;**87**(8):602-607. DOI: 10.1111/josh.12530

[47] Groffik D, Mitas J, Jakubec L, Svozil Z, Fromel K. Adolescents' physical activity in education systems varying in the number of weekly physical education lessons. Research Quarterly for Exercise and Sport. 2020;**91**(4):551-561. DOI: 10.1080/02701367.2019.1688754

[48] Sallis JF, McKenzie TL, Beets MW, Beighle A, Erwin H, Lee S. Physical education's role in public health: Steps forward and backward over 20 years and HOPE for the future. Research Quarterly for Exercise and Sport. 2012;**83**(2):125-135. DOI: 10.1080/02701367.2012.10599842

[49] Mersh R, Fairclough SJ. Physical activity, lesson context and teacher behaviours within the revised English National Curriculum for physical education: A case study of one school. European Physical Education Review. 2010;**16**(1):29-45. DOI: 10.1177/1356336X10369199

[50] McKenzie TL, Lounsbery MA. Physical education teacher effectiveness in a public health context. Research Quarterly for Exercise and Sport. 2013;**84**(4):419-430. DOI: 10.1080/02701367.2013.844025

[51] Haerens L, Kirk D, Cardon G, De Bourdeaudhuij I. Toward the development of a pedagogical model for health-based physical education. Quest. 2011;**63**(3):321-338. DOI: Doi 10.1080/00336297.2011.10483684

[52] Deci EL, Ryan RM. The "what" and "why" of goal pursuits: Human needs and the self-determination of behavior. Psychological Inquiry. 2000;**11**(4):227-268. DOI: Doi 10.1207/S15327965pli1104_01

[53] Mouratidis A, Vansteenkiste M, Lens W, Sideridis G. The motivating role of positive feedback in sport and physical education: Evidence for a motivational model. Journal of Sport & Exercise Psychology. 2008;**30**(2):240-268. DOI: 10.1123/jsep.30.2.240

[54] Phillips SR, Marttinen R, Mercier K. Fitness assessment: Recommendations for an enjoyable student experience. Strategies. 2017;**30**:19-24

Chapter 4

Assessment of Autonomic Cardiac Activity in Athletes

Júlio Costa and Fábio Y. Nakamura

Abstract

Athletes, coaches, and supporting staff should assume a scientific approach to both designing and monitoring training programs. Proper load monitoring is essential to determine whether an athlete is adapting to a training program and to minimize the risk of increasing non-functional overreaching, illness, or injury. To gain an understanding of training and competition demands and their effects on the athlete, various potential physiological variables are available. Nonetheless, very few of them have robust scientific evidence to support their use. Therefore, this chapter will discuss the use of non-invasive and time-efficient methods to record and/or calculate heart rate variability (HRV) in athletes. HRV variables can provide detailed information about positive and negative adaptions over short and long periods throughout the competitive season. The accumulated knowledge regarding the importance of HRV has led both monitoring variables to become popular strategies among elite athletes, coaches, and supporting staff.

Keywords: autonomic nervous system, heart rate variability, overnight, overload, recovery

1. Introduction

Advances in technology available for monitoring athletes has led to greater opportunities to scientifically support athletes, and, thus, information regarding the modern (elite) male and female athletes are increasingly available. Over the years, numerous techniques have been used to determine the physical and physiological profiles of athletes [1–4]. Nevertheless, for some athletes and/or teams, lacking of funds can be a main cause for not including a system of training and match workload monitoring.

However, there is increasing interest in monitoring the status of the autonomic nervous system (ANS) via measures of heart rate (HR), which includes the level but mostly focuses on the variability in HR at rest [5, 6], during exercise [7–10], and following exercise [8, 9, 11, 12]. The main interest in heart rate variability (HRV) measures is that they are non-invasive, relatively low-priced, time-efficient, and can be applied routinely and simultaneously in many athletes (i.e., in individual and team sports). While the collection of HRV (beat-by-beat) was initially only possible with expensive laboratory-based electrocardiograph recorders, the recent availability of valid and portable recorders such as HR monitors [13–24], specifically-designed systems [25, 26], or smartphone applications [27] has substantially boosted the use of HRV monitoring in the field. However, despite its common implementation in the field, the usefulness of HRV indices is still a matter of debate. While the majority of studies have shown that these measures are sensitive to fitness improvements, fatigue, overload, or detraining [28–32], others have not [5].

Therefore, this chapter will discuss the use of non-invasive and time-efficient methods to record and/or calculate HRV in athletes. HRV variables can provide detailed information about positive and negative adaptions over short and long periods throughout the competitive season. The accumulated knowledge regarding the importance of HRV has led both monitoring variables to become popular strategies among elite athletes, coaches, and supporting staff. Moreover, monitoring health parameters in athletes is also crucial to understand responses to training and readiness, enabling appropriate planning. Importantly, health monitoring also intends to reduce the risk of injury, illness, and non-functional overreaching. In addition, health status data may be useful for team selection and determining which athletes are ready to sustain competition demands.

2. The autonomic cardiac activity

Cardiovascular function is regulated by the ANS [33]. The main objective of autonomic cardiovascular regulation is to control cardiac output and the distribution of blood at the central and peripheral levels. HR and the contractile properties of the myocardium, are modulated by the main components of ANS: the parasympathetic and sympathetic nervous systems [33]. The activity of these two ANS branches with opposite effects on HR causes continuous fluctuations in HR, which is called HRV [33]. The most evident fluctuations of HR are associated to respiration and result as increased HR during inspiration and decreased HR during expiration [33].

The physiological determinants of resting HRV are multiple and include cardiac muscle morphology, plasma volume, central autonomic modulation, age, and body position [34–37]. Under normal conditions, the conduction process begins in a particular area of the heart, named the atrial sinus node, whose electrical properties can generate the action potential that spreads quickly through specialized fibres to the heart, resulting in contraction of the entire cardiac muscle [38]. In addition to this intrinsic mechanism that determines the basal cardiac rhythm, the ANS plays an important role in controlling the heart function and vascular system through the sympathetic and parasympathetic fibres to the heart, and through the sympathetic fibres to the vessels [33]. The two branches of the ANS, i.e., the sympathetic and parasympathetic fibres, act in an opposite way, providing fine adjustment to the cardiac tissues in response to different stimuli and daily activities. However, an imbalance between sympathetic and parasympathetic drives has been proposed as a potential mechanism in some cardiovascular diseases such as arterial hypertension, heart failure, and myocardial infarction [39].

3. Assessment of autonomic cardiac activity

In sports, HRV might provide useful markers of positive and negative adaptations to training and competitions [5, 40]. The basic principle of HRV monitoring is to make inferences on possible changes in cardiac ANS status due to exercise while using repeated HRV measures over time. Since ANS activity is highly sensitive to environmental conditions (e.g., noise, light, temperature) [34], it is important to take some precautions so as to standardize recording conditions, in order to isolate the training-induced effects on ANS.

Precise detection of electrocardiogram (ECG) R-waves is necessary for the analysis of beat-to-beat R-R interval oscillation [33]. In fact, for practical reasons, heart period is normally measured from R-R intervals [41]. P-R interval varies normally 120–200 ms during the Holter recording but is linearly related to R-R interval in healthy subjects. P-R interval seems to be controlled by ANS and fluctuates similarly to R-R interval [41].

The analysis in the time domain further provides other related measures, including the square root of the mean of the sum of the squares of differences between successive R–R intervals (RMSSD) and the standard deviation of the R–R intervals (SDNN) [33].

In addition, R-R interval fluctuations as a function of frequency [41, 42]. Parametric autoregressive modelling and nonparametric fast Fourier transform are the most frequently used frequency domain methods generating R-R interval power spectra [41]. R-R interval power spectra are usually divided into four bands: high-frequency (HF, 0.15–0.4 Hz), low-frequency (LF, 0.04–0.15 Hz), very-low-frequency (VLF 0.0033–0.04 Hz) and ultra-low-frequency bands (< 0.0033 Hz). The spectral power densities for VLF and ultra-low-frequency power can be reliably analyzed only from long-term recordings (> 18 hours). Power spectral densities are calculated for each band, which determines the distribution R-R interval oscillation over different frequencies [41].

Moreover, HF spectral power aims to quantify respiratory sinus arrhythmia (RSA), since spontaneous respiration frequency is commonly between the frequencies of 0.15 to 0.4 Hz [41, 42]. To ensure the presence of an evident peak within the HF band and to control the effects of respiration on HF power, a standardized respiratory pattern has been used in laboratory conditions [41, 42]. Since RSA is generated by cardiac vagal nerve traffic, HF power is considered an index of cardiac vagal outflow [41, 42]. In addition, it is important to note that HF power is the most frequently used measure to quantify vagally mediated beat-to-beat R-R interval variability [41].

Furthermore, the HF component has been widely emphasized as an index that reflects the vagal modulation, whereas the LF component reflects an interaction between sympathetic and parasympathetic modulation [43]. On the other hand, experimental data suggest that the rhythm pattern of VLF is intrinsically generated by the heart and that its oscillation is modulated by sympathetic nerve endings [44]. It is important to note that circadian rhythms, core body temperature, metabolism, hormones, and intrinsic rhythms generated by the heart all contribute to lower frequency rhythms [i.e., VLF) [38]. Moreover, long-term regulation mechanisms and ANS activity related to thermoregulation, the renin-angiotensin system, and other hormonal factors may contribute to this band [45, 46]. For instance, lower power in this band has been associated with high inflammation in a number of studies [47, 48] and has been correlated with low levels of testosterone, while higher VLF power that occurs during the night and peaks before waking have been associated with other stress biochemical markers, such as cortisol [49, 50]. In fact, authors [49] suggest that increased autonomic activity (i.e., higher VLF power) may correlate with the morning cortisol peak.

Although the ratio between LF and HF (LF/HF) has been used historically as a measure involving the sympathetic/parasympathetic balance [51], recent studies suggest that this measure cannot be used as an accurate measure of this balance [42].

4. Suggested methods for the assessment of autonomic cardiac activity

Assessment of the HRV from linear methods can be executed from records with durations of 2, 5, and 15 minutes (short-time), and over 24-hours (long-time) [18, 33]. Vagal indices of HRV, such as the logarithm RMSSD (lnRMSSD), reflecting cardiac parasympathetic modulation, are sensitive to fatigue and have been practical in evaluating individual training adaptation in team sports athletes [52, 53]. Moreover, the weekly (across 4–7 days) coefficient of variation (CV) of lnRMSSD ($lnRMSSD_{CV}$) may provide valuable information concerning training-induced perturbations in homeostasis, i.e., can reflect the day-to-day variations in cardiac parasympathetic activity [52, 54]. In general, athletes with a lower $lnRMSSD_{CV}$ present higher aerobic fitness and seem to cope better with training and match loads [55–57]. In fact, higher $lnRMSSD_{CV}$ associated with reduced average lnRMSSD during training and matches may be interpreted as a sign of overload.

Recordings of at least 2 minutes are adequate for most HRV analyses quantifying the short-term fluctuation of R-R intervals, but 5 minutes is preferable [41]. The reproducibility of short-term HRV analysis has been assessed in several ways and noted to be relatively good if measurement is highly controlled [41]. Both respiration frequency and tidal volumes affect respiratory-related R-R interval fluctuation [41]. A higher breathing rate leads to minor RSA, as a higher tidal volume increases RSA. Diurnal variation of R-R interval fluctuation [41] and a previous meal also influence short-term HRV measurements [41]. Furthermore, laboratory conditions involve some sensitive psychosomatic factors, which appear to influence the measurements [41].

The assessment of long-term 24-hour ambulatory R-R interval oscillations has been introduced as a method for the quantification of cardiac autonomic modulation [18]. The finding of an association between 24-hour HRV and mortality among patients with recent myocardial infarction increased the use of ambulatory recording for the assessment of cardiac autonomic tone [18]. The analysis of 24-hour HRV has high reproducibility with no placebo effect, and it is not dependent on the subject's cooperation [41]. The main limitation of 24-hour ambulatory R-R interval recordings is normally the uncontrolled daily activity and respiration. Despite the good reproducibility of 24-h recording., the individual differences in daily activity and respiration pattern may limit the analysis of ambulatory HRV in cross-sectional studies [18].

The presence of noise, trends, ectopic beats, and artefacts has been considered as the main problem found in records of HRV. These issues can directly affect the quality of HRV analysis, requiring signal correction [58]. Therefore, ectopic beats are, in general, automatically removed and replaced with interpolated adjacent R–R interval values using a low filter [59]. In addition, to reduce any potential non-uniformity or skewness in HRV, data can be log-transformed by taking the natural logarithm [60] before conducting any statistical analyses [31].

It is also important to note that monitoring training-related cardiac autonomic responses has been facilitated by using after-waking ultra-short-term HRV measurements in male and female athletes [61–63]. However, this method does not allow evaluation of the time course of post-exercise quantification of HRV during periods of more steady physiological states [55, 64]. Thus, HRV recordings conducted during night sleep could be an interesting substitute.

HRV data collected during selected slow-wave sleep episodes (SWSE; defined as deep stage of sleep), which offers great signal stability and high standardization of both environmental factors and respiratory influences on HRV, might be preferred [65, 66]. Nevertheless, night recordings could be difficult to implement daily [63], limiting their usefulness. Throughout the SWSE method, it was possible to observed that a single session of supramaximal intermittent exercise triggered a decrease in vagally-mediated HRV indices in young non-athletes during sleep following exercise [64]. Importantly, the SWSE requires the analysis of 10 min out of many hours of sleep.

The SWSE considers the following steps:

1. the first 10 min of the first low and regular HR episode lasting at least 15 min;

2. the lowest SDNN throughout the period of interest;

3. a circular Poincaré plot (i.e., a round cluster of points in R–R intervals plotted as a function of the previous one);

4. a low inter-beat autocorrelation between successive R–R intervals (i.e., correlation coefficient of the Poincaré plot <0.5).

In contrast, has been proposed the analyses of overnight sleep cardiac autonomic activity using an "hour-by-hour" approach using all the R–R intervals recorded throughout the sleep period [67]. The authors found that vigorous late-night exercise did not disturb sleep quality in physically active male subjects [67].

5. Conclusions

Overall, monitoring HRV in athletes can be useful for early detection and intervention before significant performance and health decrements are observed. Non-invasive and time-efficient methods/equipment such as wearable beat-to-beat HR monitors can provide detailed information about positive and negative adaptions over short and long periods throughout the competitive season. In addition, each athlete could perform the recordings at home, adopting a "real world scenario" to grant high ecological validity to the research and/or practical interventions. The accumulated knowledge regarding the importance of HRV has led HRV monitoring to become a popular strategy among elite athletes, coaches, and supporting staff.

Conflict of interest

The authors declare no conflict of interest.

Author details

Júlio Costa[1*] and Fábio Y. Nakamura[2]

1 Portugal Football School, Portuguese Football Federation (FPF), Oeiras, Portugal

2 Research Center in Sports Sciences, Health Sciences and Human Development (CIDESD), University of Maia (ISMAI), Maia, Portugal

*Address all correspondence to: jahdc@hotmail.com

References

[1] Di Salvo V, Baron R, Tschan H, Calderon Montero FJ, Bachl N, Pigozzi F. Performance characteristics according to playing position in elite soccer. International Journal of Sports Medicine. 2007;**28**(3):222-227

[2] Casamichana D, Castellano J, Castagna C. Comparing the physical demands of friendly matches and small-sided games in semiprofessional soccer players. The Journal of Strength and Conditioning Research. 2012;**26**(3):837-843

[3] Mallo J, Navarro E. Physical load imposed on soccer players during small-sided training games. The Journal of Sports Medicine and Physical Fitness. 2008;**48**(2):166-171

[4] Halson SL. Monitoring training load to understand fatigue in athletes. Sports Medicine. 2014;**44**(Suppl. 2): S139-S147

[5] Plews DJ, Laursen PB, Stanley J, Kilding AE, Buchheit M. Training adaptation and heart rate variability in elite endurance athletes: Opening the door to effective monitoring. Sports Medicine. 2013;**43**(9):773-781

[6] Stanley J, Peake JM, Buchheit M. Cardiac parasympathetic reactivation following exercise: Implications for training prescription. Sports Medicine. 2013;**43**(12):1259-1277

[7] Rowsell GJ, Coutts AJ, Reaburn P, Hill-Haas S. Effects of cold-water immersion on physical performance between successive matches in high-performance junior male soccer players. Journal of Sports Sciences. 2009;**27**(6):565-573

[8] Buchheit M, Chivot A, Parouty J, Mercier D, Al Haddad H, Laursen PB, et al. Monitoring endurance running performance using cardiac parasympathetic function. European Journal of Applied Physiology. 2010;**108**(6):1153-1167

[9] Buchheit M, Simpson MB, Al Haddad H, Bourdon PC, Mendez-Villanueva A. Monitoring changes in physical performance with heart rate measures in young soccer players. European Journal of Applied Physiology. 2012;**112**(2):711-723

[10] Garvican LA, Hammond K, Varley MC, Gore CJ, Billaut F, Aughey RJ. Lower running performance and exacerbated fatigue in soccer played at 1600 m. International Journal of Sports Physiology and Performance. 2014;**9**(3):397-404

[11] Buchheit M, Millet GP, Parisy A, Pourchez S, Laursen PB, Ahmaidi S. Supramaximal training and postexercise parasympathetic reactivation in adolescents. Medicine and Science in Sports and Exercise. 2008;**40**(2):362-371

[12] Buchheit M, Racinais S, Bilsborough JC, Bourdon PC, Voss SC, Hocking J, et al. Monitoring fitness, fatigue and running performance during a pre-season training camp in elite football players. Journal of Science and Medicine in Sport. 2013;**16**(6):550-555

[13] Parak J, Korhonen I. Accuracy of Firstbeat BodyGuard 2 beat-to-beat heart rate monitor 2015. Available from: https://www.firstbeat.com/app/uploads/2015/10/white_paper_bodyguard2_final.pdf. [Accessed: May 8, 2017]

[14] Gamelin FX, Berthoin S, Bosquet L. Validity of the polar S810 heart rate monitor to measure R-R intervals at rest. Medicine and Science in Sports and Exercise. 2006;**38**(5):887-893

[15] Weippert M, Kumar M, Kreuzfeld S, Arndt D, Rieger A, Stoll R. Comparison of three mobile devices for measuring R-R intervals and heart rate variability: Polar S810i, Suunto t6 and an ambulatory ECG system. European Journal of Applied Physiology. 2010;**109**(4):779-786

[16] Wallen MB, Hasson D, Theorell T, Canlon B, Osika W. Possibilities and limitations of the polar RS800 in measuring heart rate variability at rest. European Journal of Applied Physiology. 2012;**112**(3):1153-1165

[17] Costa J, Figueiredo P, Nakamura F, Rago V, Rebelo A, Brito J. Intra-individual variability of sleep and nocturnal cardiac autonomic activity in elite female soccer players during an international tournament. PLoS One. 2019;**14**(9):1-19

[18] Costa JA, Brito J,Nakamura FY, Dores H, Rebelo A. Associationsbetween 24- h heart rate variability and aerobic fitnessin high- level female soccer players. Scandinavian Journal of Medicine & Science in Sports. 2022;**32**(Suppl. 1):140-149. DOI: 10.1111/sms.14116

[19] Costa JA, Brito J, Nakamura FY, Figueiredo P, Oliveira E, Rebelo A. Sleep patterns and nocturnal cardiac autonomic activity in female athletes are affected by the timing of exercise and match location. Chronobiology International. 2019;**36**(3):360-373

[20] Costa JA, Brito J, Nakamura FY, Figueiredo P, Rebelo A. Using the rating of perceived exertion and heart rate to quantify training intensity in female soccer players: Validity and utility. Journal of Strength Condensed Research. 2019

[21] Costa JA, Brito J, Nakamura FY, Oliveira EM, Costa OP, Rebelo AN. Does night-training load affect sleep patterns and nocturnal cardiac autonomic activity in high-level female soccer players? International Journal of Sports Physiology and Performance. 2018;**14**(6):779-787

[22] Costa JA, Brito J, Nakamura FY, Oliveira EM, Rebelo AN. Effects of late-night training on "slow-wave sleep episode" and hour-by-hour-derived nocturnal cardiac autonomic activity in female soccer players. International Journal of Sports Physiology and Performance. 2018;**13**(5):638-644

[23] Costa JA, Figueiredo P, Nakamura FY, Rebelo A, Brito J. Monitoring individual sleep and nocturnal heart rate variability indices: The impact of training and match schedule and load in high-level female soccer players. Frontiers in Physiology. 2021;**12**:678

[24] Figueiredo P, Costa J, Lastella M, Morais J, Brito J. Sleep indices and cardiac autonomic activity responses during an international tournament in a Youth National Soccer Team. International Journal of Environmental Research and Public Health. 2021;**18**:336

[25] Parrado E, Garcia MA, Ramos J, Cervantes JC, Rodas G, Capdevila L. Comparison of omega wave system and polar S810i to detect R-R intervals at rest. International Journal of Sports Medicine. 2010;**31**(5):336-341

[26] Cassirame J, Stuckey MI, Sheppard F, Tordi N. Accuracy of the Minicardio system for heart rate variability analysis compared to ECG. The Journal of Sports Medicine and Physical Fitness. 2013;**53**(3):248-254

[27] Flatt AA, Esco MR. Validity of the ithlete Smart Phone Application for

determining ultra-short-term heart rate variability. Journal of Human Kinetics. 2013;**39**:85-92

[28] Flatt AA, Hornikel B, Esco MR. Heart rate variability and psychometric responses to overload and tapering in collegiate sprint-swimmers. Journal of Science and Medicine in Sport. 2017;**20**(6):606-610

[29] Flatt AA, Esco MR, Nakamura FY, Plews DJ. Interpreting daily heart rate variability changes in collegiate female soccer players. Journal of Sports Medicine and Physical Fitness. 2017;**57**(6):907-915

[30] Flatt AA, Esco MR, Nakamura FY. Individual heart rate variability responses to preseason training in high level female soccer players. Journal of Strength and Conditioning Research. 2017;**31**(2):531-538

[31] Mourot L, Bouhaddi M, Perrey S, Cappelle S, Henriet MT, Wolf JP, et al. Decrease in heart rate variability with overtraining: Assessment by the Poincare plot analysis. Clinical Physiology and Functional Imaging. 2004;**24**(1):10-18

[32] Pereira LA, Nakamura FY, Castilho C, Kitamura K, Kobal R, Cal Abad CC, et al. The impact of detraining on cardiac autonomic function and specific endurance and muscle power performances of high-level endurance runners. The Journal of Sports Medicine and Physical Fitness. 2016;**56**(12):1583-1591

[33] Ferreira M Jr, Zanesco A. Heart rate variability as important approach for assessment autonomic modulation. Motriz: Revista de Educação Física. 2016;**22**(2):3-8

[34] Achten J, Jeukendrup AE. Heart rate monitoring: Applications and limitations. Sports Medicine. 2003;**33**(7):517-538

[35] Aubert AE, Seps B, Beckers F. Heart rate variability in athletes. Sports Medicine. 2003;**33**(12):889-919

[36] Sandercock GR, Brodie DA. The use of heart rate variability measures to assess autonomic control during exercise. Scandinavian Journal of Medicine & Science in Sports. 2006;**16**(5):302-313

[37] Bosquet L, Merkari S, Arvisais D, Aubert AE. Is heart rate a convenient tool to monitor over-reaching? A systematic review of the literature. British Journal of Sports Medicine. 2008;**42**(9):709-714

[38] Shaffer F, McCraty R, Zerr CL. A healthy heart is not a metronome: An integrative review of the heart's anatomy and heart rate variability. Frontiers in Psychology. 2014;**5**:1040

[39] Berntson GG, Norman GJ, Hawkley LC, Cacioppo JT. Cardiac autonomic balance versus cardiac regulatory capacity. Psychophysiology. 2008;**45**:643

[40] Halson SL. Sleep in elite athletes and nutritional interventions to enhance sleep. Sports Medicine. 2014;**44**:S13

[41] TaskForce. Heart rate variability: Standards of measurement, physiological interpretation, and clinical use: Task Force of the European Society of Cardiology and the North American Society of Pacing and Eletrophysiology. European Heart Journal. 1996;**17**(3): 354-381

[42] Billman GE. The LF/HF ratio does not accurately measure cardiac sympatho-vagal balance. Frontiers in Physiology. 2013;**4**:26

[43] Kleiger RE, Stein PK, Bigger JT. Heart rate variability: Measurement and clinical utility. Annals of Noninvasive Electrocardiology. 2005;**10**(1):88-101

[44] McCraty R, Shaffer F. Heart rate variability: New perspectives on physiological mechanisms, assessment of self-regulatory capacity, and health risk. Global Advances in Health and Medicine. 2015;**4**(1):46-61

[45] Akselrod S, Gordon D, Ubel FA, Shannon DC, Berger AC, Cohen RJ. Power spectrum analysis of heart rate fluctuation: A quantitative probe of beat-to-beat cardiovascular control. Science. 1981;**213**(4504):220-222

[46] Claydon VE, Krassioukov AV. Clinical correlates of frequency analyses of cardiovascular control after spinal cord injury. American Journal of Physiology. Heart and Circulatory Physiology. 2008;**294**(2):H668-H678

[47] Carney RM, Freedland KE, Stein PK, Miller GE, Steinmeyer B, Rich MW, et al. Heart rate variability and markers of inflammation and coagulation in depressed patients with coronary heart disease. Journal of Psychosome Research. 2007;**62**(4):463-467

[48] Lampert R, Bremner JD, Su S, Miller A, Lee F, Cheema F, et al. Decreased heart rate variability is associated with higher levels of inflammation in middle-aged men. American Heart Journal. 2008;**156**(4):759

[49] Singh RB, Cornelissen G, Weydahl A, Schwartzkopff O, Katinas G, Otsuka K, et al. Circadian heart rate and blood pressure variability considered for research and patient care. International Journal of Cardiology. 2003;**87**(1):9-28

[50] Huikuri HV, Niemela MJ, Ojala S, Rantala A, Ikaheimo MJ, Airaksinen KE. Circadian rhythms of frequency domain measures of heart rate variability in healthy subjects and patients with coronary artery disease. Effects of arousal and upright posture. Circulation. 1994;**90**(1):121-126

[51] Pagani M, Lombardi F, Guzzetti S, Rimoldi O, Furlan R, Pizzinelli P, et al. Power spectral analysis of heart rate and arterial pressure variabilities as a marker of sympatho-vagal interaction in man and conscious dog. Circulation. 1986;**59**(2):178-193

[52] Buchheit M. Monitoring training status with HR measures: Do all roads lead to Rome? Frontier in Physiology. 2014;**5**:73

[53] de Freitas VH, Pereira LA, de Souza EA, Leicht AS, Bertollo M, Nakamura FY. Sensitivity of the Yo-Yo intermittent recovery test and cardiac autonomic responses to training in futsal players. International Journal of Sports Physiology and Performance. 2015;**10**(5):553-558

[54] Nakamura FY, Antunes P, Nunes C, Costa JA, Esco MR, Travassos B. Heart rate variability changes from traditional vs. ultra–short-term recordings in relation to preseason training load and performance in futsal players. Journal of Strength Condensed Research. 2018;**xx**:153

[55] Boullosa DA, Abreu L, Nakamura FY, Munoz VE, Dominguez E, Leicht AS. Cardiac autonomic adaptations in elite Spanish soccer players during preseason. International Journal of Sports Physiology and Performance. 2013;**8**(4):400-409

[56] Buchheit M, Mendez-Villanueva A, Quod MJ, Poulos N, Bourdon P. Determinants of the variability of heart rate measures during a competitive period in young soccer players. European Journal of Applied Physiology. 2010;**109**(5):869-878

[57] Flatt AA, Esco MR. Evaluating individual training adaptation with smartphone-derived heart rate variability in a collegiate female soccer team. Journal of Strength and Conditioning Research. 2016;**30**(2):378-385

[58] Huikuri HV, Makikallio T, Airaksinen KE, Mitrani R, Castellanos A, Myerburg RJ. Measurement of heart rate variability: A clinical tool or a research toy? Journal of the American College of Cardiology. 1999;**34**(7):1878-1883

[59] Tarvainen MP, Niskanen JP, Lipponen JA, Ranta-Aho PO, Karjalainen PA. Heart rate variability analysis software. Computer Methods and Programs in Biomedicine. 2014;**113**(1):210-220

[60] Ohlsson A, Berg L, Ljungberg H, Söderman K, Stålnacke B. Heart rate distribution during training and a domestic league game in swedish elite female soccer players. Annals of Sports Medicine and Research. 2015;**2**(4):1025

[61] Esco MR, Flatt AA, Nakamura FY. Initial weekly HRV response is related to the prospective change in vo2max in female soccer players. International Journal of Sports Medicine. 2016;**37**(6):436-441

[62] Fazackerley LA, Fell JW, Kitic CM. The effect of an ultra-endurance running race on heart rate variability. European Journal of Applied Physiology. 2019;**119**(9):2001-2009

[63] Stanley J, Peake JM, Buchheit M. Consecutive days of cold water immersion: Effects on cycling performance and heart rate variability. European Journal of Applied Physiology. 2013;**113**(2):371-384

[64] Al Haddad H, Laursen PB, Ahmaidi S, Buchheit M. Nocturnal heart rate variability following supramaximal intermittent exercise. International Journal of Sports Physiology and Performance. 2009;**4**(4):435-447

[65] Brandenberger G, Buchheit M, Ehrhart J, Simon C, Piquard F. Is slow wave sleep an appropriate recording condition for heart rate variability analysis? Autonomic Neuroscience. 2005;**121**(1-2):81-86

[66] Buchheit M, Simon C, Piquard F, Ehrhart J, Brandenberger G. Effects of increased training load on vagal-related indexes of heart rate variability: A novel sleep approach. American Journal of Physiology. Heart and Circulatory Physiology. 2004;**287**(6):H2813-H2818

[67] Myllymaki T, Kyrolainen H, Savolainen K, Hokka L, Jakonen R, Juuti T, et al. Effects of vigorous late-night exercise on sleep quality and cardiac autonomic activity. Journal of Science and Medicine in Sport. 2011;**20** (1 Pt 2):146-153

Chapter 5

Swimming Exercise-Induced Improvements in Cardiorespiratory Fitness (CRF) are Caused by Nitric Oxide Functional Adaptations in the Oxygen Transport System

Jia-Ping Wu

Abstract

Cardiorespiratory fitness (CRF) is associated with referring to enhance oxygen transport capacity to respiratory systems and increasing oxygen transport circulatory to skeletal muscle to produce energy. The aim of this report on the health-related CRF in the oxygen transport system-mediated physiological nitric oxide (NO) functional adaptations. Therefore, we want to know that swimming exercise-induced improvements in CRF resulted in increased oxygen transport capacity during physical activity of the respiratory systems. Therefore, the oxygen circulatory transport system is related to NO signaling and has been associated with various pathophysiologic functions and neuronal activity. Besides mediating normal functions, NO is implicated in inflammation and hypertension disease states. Swimming exercise is a good way to increase the rate of metabolism. Swimming exercise improves heart rate and oxygen circulatory, and increases the rate of metabolism and burning of heat. In this context, this review summarizes the roles of NO in improvements in cardiorespiratory fitness.

Keywords: cardiorespiratory fitness, nitric oxide, oxygen circulatory transport, swimming exercise, hypertension diseases states

1. Introduction

Cardiorespiratory fitness (CRF) is a measure of health in certain youth and elderly persons. Thus, CRF can be tracked and assessed time in youth and compared across populations. Although cardiorespiratory fitness (CRF) is not recommended pharmacological treatment for a broad range of diseases such as congenital heart disease, asthma, and cystic fibrosis, it is widely accepted as an intervention in exercise training and nutritional supplementation to maintain skeletal muscle mass and strength [1]. Estimating CRF is an important marker of health outcomes in youth and the elderly. CRF plays an essential role in referring to the capacity of the circulatory and respiratory systems to supply oxygen to skeletal muscle energy needed during water aerobics exercises [2]. Interestingly,

IntechOpen

a number of retrospective and prospective studies on a cohort of community-living older individuals have suggested that only 40% of the U.S. population is currently believed to have healthy CRF. CRF is one of the five health-related components of physical fitness. It differs from other components of physical fitness, including body composition, muscular strength, muscular endurance, and flexibility [3]. The assessment of CRF is an important part of the prevention and rehabilitation program. CRF is characterized by the body's ability to perform moderate- to vigorous-intensity activity using large muscle groups for prolonged periods of time [4]. Both CRF and exercise have been associated with a wide range of health outcomes achievement in youth quality of life.

With all the exercise training we face during pre-activity screening these days and pertinent data, it is essential to remember that unwanted or potentially harmful events may occur during the exercise test. Above all, if we can develop a more cost-effective CRF measurement process, we will have a better chance of delaying aging. These instructions on the exercise test should be provided to patients for at least 24 hours to ensure that their respiratory, cardiovascular, and musculoskeletal systems work together [5]. The ability to sustain this level of exertion depends on adherence to instructions as well as maximizing patient safety and comfort. Additionally, the measurement of CRF can be used as a reference for developing regular new modes for an exercise program by providing information on how to initiate the exercise training program. One of the said modes recommends an increase in intensity and duration to improve overall fitness. The following measurement of CRF can provide professionals with valuable information on the motivation for periodically screening all youth patients' regular exercise programs [6]; it can be characterized as a program setting-response relationship. Increases in CRF are associated with a number of health benefits. Higher levels of CRF are often associated with a significant increase in physical activity [7]. The measurement of CRF is typically expressed in absolute or relative terms. The absolute maximal volume of oxygen consumed per unit time (VO_{2max}, L/min, or ml/min) is expressed as a measure of energy expenditure for both non-weight-bearing and weight-bearing exercises. VO_{2max} is accepted as the criterion measure of CRF. Absolute VO_{2max} is most often described as directly relative to body mass or an individual's body size; it is typically greater in young people compared to old people. Relative VO_{2max} (ml/kg × min) is often used to estimate energy expenditure of weight-bearing exercises such as walking, running, and stair climbing when VO_{2max} is expressed as simply a linear function of body mass. As is well-known, health is definitely important in human life and work. In fact, having excessive wealth without good health is of no use for 99% of us, and a few of us will die due to poor health.

2. Aerobic swimming exercise

Adaptation of exercise plans should follow individual goals, taking aerobic exercise became restricted to swimming, walking, running, cycling, skating, riding, and all challenges. A high degree of accuracy in exercise suggestions for the elderly was achieved by applying the aerobic swimming exercise model. Therefore, there is no need to tell that good health is important for periodic assessment to ascertain how quickly the condition is improving or worsening [8]. Do you warm up before undergoing swimming training? The aerobic swimming exercise protocol consisted of warm-up exercise, real exercise, and relaxation. Based on the basic information all of them finished their own exercise intervention for elder humans, and get personalized exercise prescriptions for each rate such as frequency, intensity, time, and volume. How good is swimming as an

Physiological principles	Low grip strength	Gait speed	Low muscle mass
Exercise training	Increase	Increase	Increase
Running	No effect	Increase	Increase
Cycling	Increase	Increase	Increase
Swimming	No effect	No effect	Increase
Walking	No effect	Increase	Increase
Tai Chi	Increase	Increase	Increase
Resistance exercise	Increase	Increase	Increase

Table 1.
Any type of CRF testing is substantial overlap between the conditions, particularly with regard to physical aspects: low grip strength, gait speed, and low muscle mass.

aerobic exercise? Switching up cardiopulmonary fitness exercises is another great way to improve your cardiorespiratory fitness exercises [9]. All those activities will still give you the aerobic cardiorespiratory fitness training that you need to develop for aerobic swimming exercise [10]. If you are training to run a marathon, do not be afraid to swap out running a few days a week for biking, rowing, or even swimming. They will utilize different muscles, helping to increase your all-around endurance capacity (**Table 1**).

3. Acute pulmonary respiratory embolism

Cold-induced asthma is usually defined as a respiratory disorder characterized by sneezing, sore throat, coughing, etc. caused by how much air moves in and out as you breathe. Catching a cold is not uncommon in a human being's life, but as far as the treatment is concerned, it may vary from culture to culture, from individual, and from setting to setting [11]. Asthma, a chronic inflammatory disorder of the airways, affects 3–5% of the population in the United States and can be fatal. Acute pulmonary respiratory embolism is characterized by episodic airway narrowing and increased airway reactivity to a variety of stimuli and spontaneous reversibility. The inflammatory response involves a respiratory infection or chronic obstructive pulmonary disease (COPD). An imbalance in proinflammatory produces multiple mediators about signs and symptoms and any other health problems. Acute pulmonary respiratory embolism may be a fundamental part of the pathogenesis of asthma [12]. Acute pulmonary respiratory embolism estimates the narrowing of your bronchial tubes by checking how much air you can exhale after a deep breath and how fast can breathe out. The histologic findings in asthma are airway cellular infiltration, epithelial disruption, mucosal edema, and mucus plugging. When your airways are acute pulmonary respiratory embolism, you may have higher than normal nitric oxide (NO) levels. This test has been widely available. Acute pulmonary respiratory embolism provokes the inflammatory response may be exposure to vigorous physical activity or taking several breaths of cold air [13].

Even in people with no history of asthma, respiratory infection is occasionally associated with increased airway reactivity for several weeks to months after the resolution of the infection; some of these persons develop chronic asthma [14]. The symptoms are persistent wheezing, chronic episodic dyspnea, and chronic cough. Patients may present with only one or a combination of the foregoing symptoms [15]. Aerobic swimming exercise should be maintained, and a clear swimming exercise plan should be in place for using the information to intervene early in exacerbations and to alter long-term swimming exercise therapy for optimal control of symptoms [16]. Having acute pulmonary respiratory embolism does not mean you have to be less active. Getting aerobic swimming exercises can prevent asthma attacks and control symptoms during activity tied for additional symptomatic control as needed [17]. Regular swimming exercises can strengthen your heart and lungs, which helps relieve asthma symptoms. If you swim exercise in cold temperatures to warm the air you breathe. These exercises may reduce the amount of medication you need to keep your asthma symptoms under control [18]. Aerobic swimming exercise preparations may have additional beneficial effects on some patients, but the narrow therapeutic and modest efficacy of these preparations limit their value [19]. Acute severe asthma or status asthmaticus is an attack of severe bronchospasm that is unresponsive to routine therapy [20]. In most cases, however, patients have a history of progressive dyspnea over hours to days, with increasing bronchodilator use. The arterial blood gas analysis in patients with mild asthma attacks or early in course of a severe asthma attack shows hypoxemia (a widened alveolar-arterial oxygen gradient) and hyperventilation (a creased Pct CO2) [21]. With O2 increasing after swimming exercises and the severity of respiratory muscle fitness, the Pa CO2 returns to normal and ultimately begins to balance. A rising Pa O2 in a patient with asthma is a healthy sign [22].

4. Cardiorespiratory fitness (CRF)

WHO defines health positively as a state of complete physical, mental and social well-being and not merely the absence of disease or infirmity [23]. In other words, a person may be healthy as a human being is the extent of an individual's continuing physical strong, emotional, and mental. The cardiorespiratory fitness and social ability associated with heart failure and resistance to infection are able to cope with physical hardships to cope with his physical environment. The cardiac cycle strongly correlates with heart failure, physical inactivity, and low fitness. If this mental state still is considered unhealthy, as measured by behavior, is deemed unsound. There is a wide variable area between CRF health and heart disease [24]. Cardiorespiratory fitness (CRF) could be defined theoretically in terms of certain measured values, for example, the sensitivity of blood pressure, acuity of vision, body temperature, height, weight, a person having normal breath, etc. [25]. Cardiac arrest cycle diseases can be defined at the simplest heart disease level as any deviation from normal form and function may either be associated with illness or be latent (**Figure 1**). Some CRF experts prefer to divide the spectrum of fitness health and heart disease into normal, cardiac hypertrophy, and heart failure. During cardiorespiratory fitness improvements, a person may have a disease for many years without even being aware of its presence. Despite the fact of a person's disease and low CRF levels are often used interchangeably, low CRF level is not equated with disease. Although heart disease, this person is not ill. For example, a person with diabetes who has received adequate insulin treatment is not ill. Regrettably, many low CRF diseases escape detection and possible cure because they remain symptomless for long years before they produce discomfort or impair function (**Figure 1**). Heart failure occurs when an abnormality of cardiac function fails to provide adequate blood flow to meet the metabolic needs of the body's tissues and organs [26]. Heart failure can result from a large number of heterogeneous disorders (**Figure 1**). One of the most common causes is idiopathic cardiomyopathy, which, strictly defined, is a primary myocardial disease of unknown etiology. However, in the low CRF clinical setting, cardiomyopathy

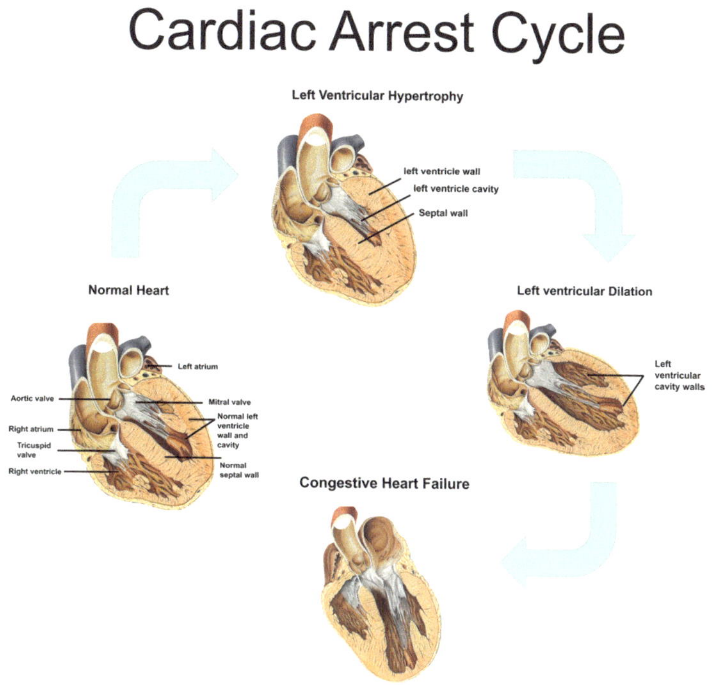

Figure 1.
Cardiac arrest cycle.

may be used to refer to myocardial dysfunction that is the result of a known cardiac systemic disease [27]. These cardiomyopathies may be related to a number of disorders. They are most often the result of ischemic heart disease. Ventricular dysfunction can also result from excessive pressure overloads, long-standing hypertension, aortic stenosis, and volume overloads (**Figure 2**). Cardiac systemic diseases that result in infiltration and replacement of normal myocardial tissue, such as amyloidosis and hemochromatosis can result in both abnormal ventricular filling as well as emptying. Diseases of the pericardium, such as chronic pericarditis or pericardial tamponade, can impair cardiac function without directly affecting the myocardial tissue. Long-standing tachyarrhythmias have been associated with myocardial dysfunction, especially in children. In addition, an individual with underlying myocardial or valvular disease will often develop heart failure with the acute onset of an arrhythmia. Finally, there are multiple metabolic abnormalities (thiamine deficiency, thyrotoxicosis), drugs (alcohol, doxorubicin), and toxic chemicals (lead, cobalt) that can impair cardiac performance. The history and physical examination are an integral part of the diagnosis of heart failure and in the determination of its underlying or precipitating use [28].

The cardiac cycle is a series of pressure changes that take place within the heart. Cardiac hypertrophy is a related change in cardiac morphology, including a decrease in myocyte number, an increase in myocyte size, a decrease in matrix connective tissue, an increase in left ventricular wall thickness, a decrease in conduction fiber density, and a decrease in sinus node cell number.

One of the cardinal manifestations of left ventricular heart failure is dyspnea, which is related to elevation in pulmonary venous pressure resulting in acute pulmonary respiratory embolism. In patients with chronic heart failure, shortness of breath initially occurs with exertion but may progress to occur at acute pulmonary

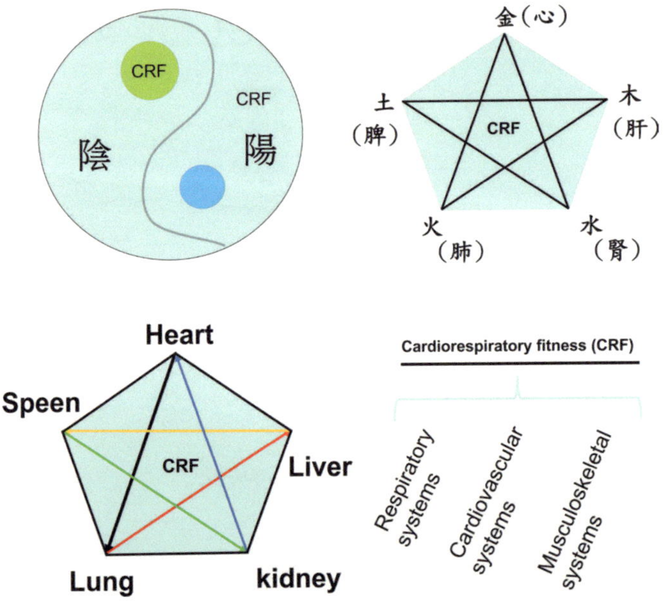

Figure 2.
The ability of yin and yang to sustain cardiorespiratory fitness level of exertion is dependent on the integration of the respiratory, cardiovascular, and musculoskeletal systems.

respiratory embolism. Cardiac dyspnea is often worsened by the recumbent position when increased venous return further elevates pulmonary respiratory embolism [29]. If heart failure is predominantly systolic with low cardiac output, the patient may complain primarily of pulmonary respiratory embolism due to diminished blood flow to the exercising muscles. In some exercise training, heart failure is slow to progress and the patient may unknowingly restrict his or her activities [30]. Thus, the history should not only include an assessment of the patient's symptoms but also the level of functional capacity. Many patients will complain of peripheral pulmonary respiratory embolism. Many aerobic swimming exercise findings of heart failure are related to the neurohormonal changes that help compensate for the reduced cardiac output and acute pulmonary respiratory embolism [31]. An increased CRF may be present as a result of decreased sympathetic tone. If left ventricular fining pressures are elevated, breath broken may be heard during auscultation of the lung fields. Acute pulmonary respiratory embolism may reveal left ventricular enlargement. A third heart sound is consistent with systolic dysfunction and can be generated from the left or right ventricle [32]. A fourth heart sound suggests a noncompliant ventricle but is not specific for heart failure. The murmurs of both mitral and tricuspid regurgitation are common in patients with congestive heart failure and may become accentuated during an acute decompensation. As acute pulmonary respiratory embolism earlier, lung edema is related to elevation in venous pressure and/or increased sodium and water retention. In low CRF patients, the edema may predominantly be in the lung region. The electrocardiogram in patients with congestive heart failure is not specific, but it may provide insight into the etiology of the cardiac dysfunction, such as prior myocardial infarction, left ventricular hypertrophy, or significant arrhythmias [33]. The chest radiograph may show chamber enlargement and signs of pulmonary congestion. Treatment of heart failure will rest on the improvement of vascular congestion on the chest radiograph, but these changes maybe 24–48 hours behind clinical improvement. Certain CRF levels may be altered in patients with heart failure [34]. The serum sodium concentration may be low, owing to increased water retention with activation of the renin-angiotensin system. Renal function may be impaired secondary to intrinsic kidney disease and/or reduced perfusion secondary to renal artery vasoconstriction and low cardiac output. Hepatic congestion is common with right-sided heart failure and may result in elevated liver enzyme levels (**Figure 2**). Because many of the signs and symptoms of heart failure may also occur with pulmonary disease, differentiating between these two disease processes may be difficult [35]. Initial therapy will often be directed at both potential pulmonary and cardiac causes until further testing can be performed. In addition, pulmonary edema may be secondary to noncardiac causes, such as severe infection, drug toxicity, or neurologic jury. This syndrome termed adult respiratory distress syndrome (ARDS), can be differentiated from cardiogenic pulmonary edema by the presence of a low or normal pulmonary capillary wedge pressure [36].

5. Cardiorespiratory fitness (CRF) in elderly people

Cardiorespiratory fitness in men and women decreases at a nonlinear rate with age. However, CRF in adults is influenced by lifestyle. Low CRF is associated with the risk of diseases that accelerates after 45 years of age and the ability of older persons to function independently. The association of aging is a lifestyle with CRF decline. The assessment of CRF can assist in identifying how to maintain a low BMI and in diagnosing whether or not an individual has been physically active. Not smoking is associated with higher CRF across the adult lifespan and prognosis of comorbid conditions [37]. CRF declines as age increases in the elderly. The measurement of CRF following the initiation of an exercise training program can motivate patients to continue with a regular exercise program and may encourage them to develop other modes of exercise to improve their overall fitness. CRF may be underestimated for heavier individuals (>75.4 kg) and overestimated for lighter individuals (<67.7 kg). An individualized CRF exercise prescription can maintain the CRF level and delay the aging process. CRF refers to the ability of the circulatory and respiratory systems to supply oxygen to skeletal muscle mitochondria to generate the energy required for physical activity [38]. Tai Chi can prevent cardiovascular disease and improve the cardiopulmonary function of adults with obesity aged 50 years and older. **Figure 2** shows a long-term follow-up study. Once an individual has been properly screened and it has been determined that it is safe for him or her to undergo the CRF test, the exercise professional should ensure that the following pretest instructions are given to him or her (**Figure 2**).

The aim of the present chapter is to review the patient's completed consent and screening forms. We found the current evidence of the importance of CRF and swimming exercise therapy for the prevention and treatment of heart failure. We find CRF assessment costly, labor-intensive, and not widely available. In this paper, we review the low-grade inflammation combined with metabolic aberrations that determine CRF, the tools are promoting available to assess CRF, constituting a pathway toward the manifestation of heart failure. The modifiable and nonmodifiable factors influencing CRF, promoting vascular dysfunction and myocardial remodeling, the autonomic imbalance have been associated with CRF with markers of health in otherwise healthy elderly people subclinical cardiac dysfunction in obese individuals, and the temporal trends in CRF both in the United States and internationally. We find that BMI is used to classify an individual's CRF level to allow for meaningful comparisons between/among individuals with different body weights. In this chapter, a new

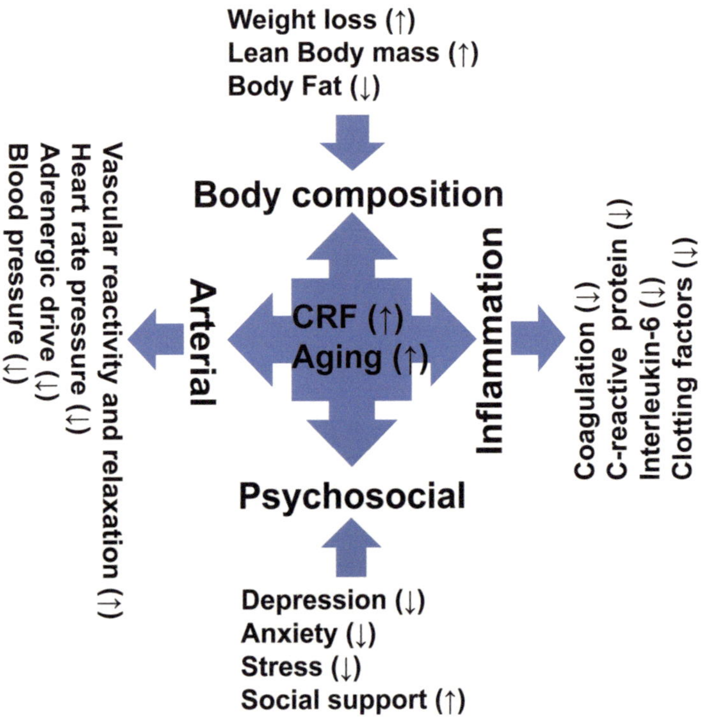

Figure 3.
The aim is to develop a new self-reported questionnaire to estimate CRF. Patient-reported outcome measures estimate CRF more cost-efficiently, but current questionnaires lack accuracy. The knowledge required to complete the assessment, interpret the results, and write an appropriate exercise prescription are an important responsibility of the exercise professional.

study based on a back-propagation (BP) neural network, is investigated to predict the individualized CRF exercise prescriptions for the elderly by correlating variables (**Figure 3**). The VO_{2max}'s expected improvement was set at 10%. The raw data are split into two parts, 90% for training the machine and the remaining 10% for testing the performance. The CRF exercise professional should be familiar with the emergency response plan. Assure a room temperature between 68 and 72°F (20 and 22°C) and a humidity of less than 60% with adequate ventilation. The testing environment can play a very important role in test validity and reliability [39]. Traditional exercise prescriptions are general and lack individualization. The definition of "long" varies according to the type of exertion—minutes for high-intensity anaerobic exercise, hours or days for low-intensity aerobic exercise [40]. It is important for the exercise professional to understand what the appropriate response to exercise is, so he or she can correctly interpret what an inappropriate BP response to exercise is.

6. NO functional adaptations in the oxygen transport system

Muscle cells carry out an increased rate of aerobic respiration to release more energy. This means the cells require more oxygen and glucose. The heart pumps faster to send more blood, containing oxygen and glucose to the cells. You also increase your breathing rate to get more oxygen into your body. The results show that the post-VO_{2max} was significantly different from the pre-VO_{2max} and improved by 10.1% [41]. The NO signaling pathway is an endogenously generated regulator of vascular via cGMP leading to smooth muscle relaxation which is the primary mechanism of NO-mediated physiology. The discovery of a signaling pathway driven by the effect of CRF level on cerebral oxygenation during exercise and cognitive tasks [42]. Indeed, it is now established the small-molecule species NO has an important physiological function, and the NO signaling pathway occurs in an integrated fashion [43]. Cardiorespiratory fitness (CRF) is defined as the peak oxygen uptake. The production of NO and cardiorespiratory fitness (CRF) can improve performance with vascular remodeling [44]. However, the probability of transitioning to more severe frailty states was much higher than the opposite way and will often lead to a spiral decline of increasing frailty and a higher risk of worsening disability, falls, hospital admissions, and death [45]. Overall, we have presented comprehensive NO functional adaptations in line with critical signaling pathways that drive the maturation of the heart during cardiorespiratory fitness (CRF).

7. Conclusion

Cardiorespiratory fitness (CRF) improvements have gained popularity over the past years. In recent years, an increasing exercise number of randomized control CRF evaluated the beneficial effects of the cardiac cycle on balance function. Some reports have reported the beneficial effects of swimming exercise on CRF in the elderly, while others' exercises have not, probably due to differences. To resolve the disparity in this book chapter review, we conducted a systematic literature review and NO functional adaptations in the oxygen transport system to elucidate the effects of swimming exercise on CRF in the elderly (**Figure 4**).

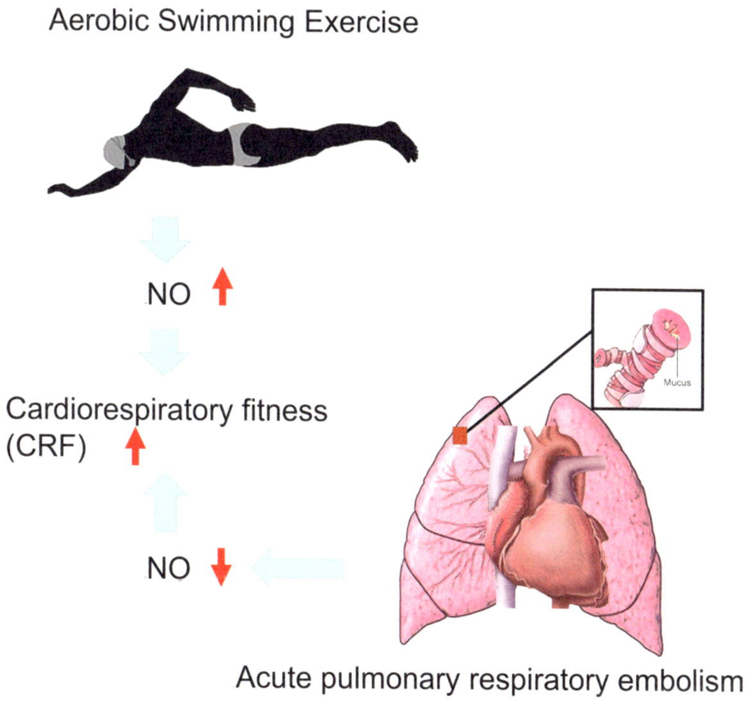

Figure 4.
A systematic literature review for cardiorespiratory fitness.

It aims to evaluate whether aerobic swimming exercise increases NO pulmonary vasodilator efficacy for acute pulmonary respiratory embolism by high-level cardiorespiratory fitness.

Author details

Jia-Ping Wu
Department of Medical Technology, Medical College of Shaoguan University, Shaoguan Guangdong Province, China PRC

*Address all correspondence to: wu20227050@163.com; wujiaping20227050@sgu.edu.cn; affymax0823@hotmail.com.tw

References

[1] Kolu P, Raitanen J, Sievänen H, Tokola K, Vähä-Ypyä H, Nieminen E, et al. Cardiorespiratory fitness is associated with sickness absence and work ability. Occupational Medicine (London). 2022;**72**:478-485

[2] Song BK, Saavedra JM, Lefferts EC, Brellenthin AG, Lee DC. Associations between cardiorespiratory fitness and diverticulitis in older adults. PLoS One. 2022;**17**:e0275433

[3] Burden SJ, Weedon BD, Turner A, Whaymand L, Meaney A, Dawes H, et al. Intensity and duration of physical activity and cardiorespiratory fitness. Pediatrics. 2022;**150**:e2021056003

[4] O'Brien MW, Mekary S, Kimmerly DS. Aging, cardiorespiratory fitness and sympathetic transduction. Aging (Albany NY). 2022;**14**:4189-4190

[5] Nagel TR, Melton BF, Keeler JM, Cross BL, Blumenburg WT, Flatt AA, et al. Cardiorespiratory fitness is inversely associated with aortic arterial stiffness in firefighters. Journal of Occupational and Environmental Medicine. 2022;**64**:e641-e646

[6] Payandeh N, Shahinfar H, Babaei N, Davarzani S, Ebaditabar M, Djafarian K, et al. Association between the empirical dietary inflammatory index and cardiorespiratory fitness in Tehranian adults in 2017-2018. Frontiers in Nutrition. 2022;**9**:928308

[7] Vesperman CJ, Wang R, Schultz SA, Law LL, Dougherty RJ, Ma Y, et al. Cardiorespiratory fitness and cognition in persons at risk for Alzheimer's disease. Alzheimer's & Dementia. 2022;**14**:e12330

[8] Mongin D, Chabert C, Extremera MG, Hue O, Courvoisier DS, Carpena P, et al. Decrease of heart rate variability during exercise: An index of cardiorespiratory fitness. PLoS One. 2022;**17**:e0273981

[9] Babity M, Zámodics M, Lakatos BK, Rákóczi R, König A, Menyhárt-Hetényi A, et al. Cardiorespiratory fitness status of elite handball referees in Hungary. PLoS One. 2022;**17**:e0270999

[10] Rose GA, Davies RG, Appadurai IR, Williams IM, Bashir M, Berg RMG, et al. "Fit for surgery": The relationship between cardiorespiratory fitness and postoperative outcomes. Experimental Physiology. 2022;**107**:787-799

[11] Michalski M, Rowed K, Lavery JA, Moskowitz CS, Capaci C, Stene G, et al. Validity of estimated cardiorespiratory fitness in patients with primary breast cancer. JACC: CardioOncology. 2022;**4**:210-219

[12] Peck SS, Esmaeilzadeh M, Rankin K, Shalmon T, Fan CS, Somerset E, et al. Self-reported physical activity, QoL, cardiac function, and cardiorespiratory fitness in women with HER2+ breast cancer. JACC: CardioOncology. 2022;**4**:387-400

[13] Kokkinos P, Faselis C, Samuel IBH, Pittaras A, Doumas M, Murphy R, et al. Cardiorespiratory fitness and mortality risk across the spectra of age, race, and sex. Journal of the American College of Cardiology. 2022;**80**:598-609

[14] Shawar RS, Puyau M, Shypailo R, Musaad S, Butte NF, Bacha F, et al. Adiposity, insulin resistance, cardiorespiratory fitness, and bone health in Hispanic children. The Journal of Clinical Endocrinology and Metabolism. 2022;**107**:e3797-e3804

[15] Mishima RS, Ariyaratnam JP, Pitman BM, Malik V, Emami M, McNamee O, et al. Cardiorespiratory fitness, obesity and left atrial function in patients with atrial fibrillation. International Journal of Cardiology. Heart & Vasculature. 2022;**42**:101083

[16] Ding Z, Du L. Swimming exercise ameliorates depressive-like behavior by anti-inflammation activity, rebalancing gut *Escherichia coli* and Lactobacilli. Brain Research. 2022;**1797**:148113

[17] Zargani M, Rahimi A, Mazaheri Tirani Z, Arabzadeh E, Feizolahi F. Swimming exercise and nano-L-arginine supplementation improve oxidative capacity and some autophagy-related genes in the soleus muscle of aging rats. Gene. 2022;**850**:146955

[18] Xie Y, Wu Z, Zhou L, Sun L, Xiao L, Wang G. Swimming exercise modulates gut microbiota in CUMS-induced depressed mice. Neuropsychiatric Disease and Treatment. 2022;**18**:749-760

[19] Song L, Mao J, Wang Q, Chen A, Sun R, Li X, et al. Long-lasting and sex-dependent effects of postweaning swimming exercise on social dominance in adult mice. Neuroscience. 2022;**498**:224-234

[20] Li G, Xu K, Xing W, Yang H, Li Y, Wang X, et al. Swimming exercise alleviates endothelial mitochondrial fragmentation via inhibiting dynamin-related protein-1 to improve vascular function in hypertension. Hypertension. 2022;**79**:e116-e128

[21] Zargani M, Hatami Nasab Z, Feizolahi F, Arabzadeh E. Swimming exercise with L-arginine coated nano-particles supplementation upregulated HAND2 and TBX5 expression in the cardiomyocytes of aging male rats. Biogerontology. 2022;**23**:473-484

[22] Catinelli BB, Rossignoli PS, Floriano JF, Carr AM, de Oliveira RG, Dos Santos NJ. Diamater study group reversal of diabetic-induced myopathy by swimming exercise in pregnant rats: A translational intervention study. Scientific Reports. 2022;**12**:7375

[23] Ebrahimian F, Najdi N, Masrour FF, Salari AA. Swimming exercise strain-dependently affects maternal care and depression-related behaviors through gestational corticosterone and brain serotonin in postpartum dams. Brain Research Bulletin. 2022;**188**:122-130

[24] Nazari M, Kordi MR, Minasian V, Quchan AHSK. Ameliorating effect of 6-week swimming exercise on mice with experimental autoimmune encephalomyelitis (EAE) by reducing fetuin-A and increasing AMPK & NAD+ levels in liver tissue. Iranian Journal of Basic Medical Sciences. 2022;**25**:1016-1020

[25] García I, Molina-Molina M, Arrillaga B, Javierre C, Viscor G. Swimming exercise for patients with long-term respiratory post COVID-19 complications: Further thinking on the pulmonary rehabilitation. Archivos de Bronconeumología. 2022;**58**:527-528

[26] da Silva Pereira MM, de Melo IMF, Braga VAÁ, Teixeira ÁAC, Wanderley-Teixeira V. Effect of swimming exercise, insulin-associated or not, on inflammatory cytokines, apoptosis, and collagen in diabetic rat placentas. Histochemistry and Cell Biology. 2022;**157**:467-479

[27] Habibi P, Ahmadiasl N, Nourazarian A, Yousefi H. Swimming exercise improves SIRT1, NF-κB, and IL-1β protein levels and pancreatic tissue injury in ovariectomized diabetic rats. Hormone Molecular Biology and Clinical Investigation. 2022;**43**:345-352

[28] Aguilar-Peralta AK, Gonzalez-Vazquez A, Tomas-Sanchez C, Blanco-Alvarez VM, Martinez-Fong D, Gonzalez-Barrios JA, et al. Prophylactic zinc administration combined with swimming exercise prevents cognitive-emotional disturbances and tissue injury following a transient hypoxic-ischemic insult in the rat. Behavioural Neurology. 2022;**2022**:5388944

[29] Hegazy MA, Abdelmonsif DA, Zeitoun TM, El-Sayed NS, Samy DM. Swimming exercise versus L-carnosine supplementation for Alzheimer's dementia in rats: Implication of circulating and hippocampal FNDC5/irisin. Journal of Physiology and Biochemistry. 2022;**78**:109-124

[30] Almeida RL, Ogihara CA, de Souza JS, Oliveira KC, Cafarchio EM, Tescaro L, et al. Regularly swimming exercise modifies opioidergic neuromodulation in rostral ventrolateral medulla in hypertensive rats. Brain Research. 2021;**1774**:147726

[31] Forte LDM, de Almeida RN, Cordeiro AV, de Fante T, de Paula Simino LA, de Souza TA, et al. Effect of acute swimming exercise at different intensities but equal total load over metabolic and molecular responses in swimming rats. Journal of Muscle Research and Cell Motility. 2022;**43**:35-44

[32] Almási G, Bosnyák E, Móra Á, Zsákai A, Fehér PV, Annár D, et al. Physiological and psychological responses to a maximal swimming exercise test in adolescent elite athletes. International Journal of Environmental Research and Public Health. 2021;**18**:9270

[33] Alomari MA, Alzoubi KH, Khabour OF. Swimming exercise improves short- and long-term memories: Time-course changes. Physiological Reports. 2021;**9**:e14851

[34] Moayeri A, Darvishi M, Hamidabadi HG, Mojaverrostami S. Potential role of human chorionic gonadotropin supplementation in spermatogenesis in rats subjected to forced swimming exercise. Folia Medica (Plovdiv). 2021;**63**:710-719

[35] Evans ML, Praebel K, Peruzzi S, Amundsen PA, Bernatchez L. Phenotype-environment association of the oxygen transport system in trimorphic European whitefish (*Coregonus lavaretus*) populations. Evolution. 2014;**68**:2197-2210

[36] Porteus CS, Wright PA, Milsom WK. The effect of sustained hypoxia on the cardio-respiratory response of bowfin Amia calva: Implications for changes in the oxygen transport system. Journal of Fish Biology. 2013;**84**:827-843

[37] Evans ML, Praebel K, Peruzzi S, Bernatchez L. Parallelism in the oxygen transport system of the lake whitefish: The role of physiological divergence in ecological speciation. Molecular Ecology. 2012;**21**:4038-4050

[38] Tiwari T, Upadhyaya DN, Dheer Y, Singh GP, Tiwari S. Formulation of an oxygen policy to ensure adequate supply of oxygen reserves during the second wave of COVID-19 pandemic. Medical Gas Research. 2023;**13**:39-40

[39] Lemke MD, Woodson JD. Targeted for destruction: Degradation of singlet oxygen-damaged chloroplasts. Plant Signaling & Behavior. 2022;**17**:2084955

[40] Wagner JM, Klok CJ, Duell ME, Socha JJ, Cao G, Gong H, et al. Isometric spiracular scaling in scarab beetles-implications for diffusive and advective oxygen transport. eLife. 2022;**11**:e82129

[41] Chen J, Liu L, Wang W, Gao H. Nitric oxide, nitric oxide formers and their physiological impacts in bacteria. International Journal of Molecular Sciences. 2022;**23**:10778

[42] Suschek CV, Feibel D, von Kohout M, Opländer C. Enhancement of nitric oxide bioavailability by modulation of cutaneous nitric oxide stores. Biomedicine. 2022;**10**:2124

[43] Soundararajan L, Dharmarajan A, Samji P. Regulation of pleiotropic physiological roles of nitric oxide signaling. Cellular Signalling. 2022;**110496**

[44] Finding EJT, Elliott J, Harris PA, Menzies-Gow NJ. Nitric oxide synthase inhibition reveals differences in the nitric oxide pathway in previously laminitic ponies. Research in Veterinary Science. 2022;**150**:79-82

[45] Lundberg JO, Weitzberg E. Nitric oxide signaling in health and disease. Cell. 2022;**185**:2853-2878

Chapter 6

The Role of Cardiorespiratory Fitness in Children with Cardiovascular Risk

Mirjam Močnik and Nataša Marčun Varda

Abstract

Cardiorespiratory fitness is an outcome of physical activity, enabling the transport of oxygen from the atmosphere to the mitochondria to perform physical work and therefore reflects the overall capacity of the cardiovascular and respiratory systems to perform the prolonged exercise. In recent decades, it has declined in the paediatric population. Cardiovascular fitness measurement has yet to be standardised in children but is a powerful marker of health in youth and is strongly associated with inflammation and inversely associated with cardiovascular risk factors, especially obesity. Notably, youth with low cardiorespiratory fitness levels have a higher risk of developing cardiovascular diseases during adulthood. Lowered cardiorespiratory fitness has been demonstrated most often in children with obesity and associated cardiovascular comorbidities, however, these can be associated with cardiorespiratory fitness independently to body mass index. The benefits of physical activity on health have been well demonstrated during growth and it should be encouraged in children with cardiovascular risk to prevent further reduction of cardiorespiratory fitness and the development of other comorbidities. Along with appropriate physical exercise and diet in childhood, breastfeeding in the first year of life is recommended.

Keywords: cardiorespiratory fitness, children, obesity, traditional cardiovascular risk, novel cardiovascular risk

1. Introduction

Cardiorespiratory fitness presents individuals' ability to transport oxygen from the atmosphere to the mitochondria to perform physical work and therefore reflects the overall capacity of the cardiovascular and respiratory systems to perform prolonged exercise [1]. Cardiovascular fitness is therefore reflected in the ability of physical activity, which is critical in childhood as it lays the foundations for later physical activity – the base on which children can build more specific motor skills or develop movement patterns [2].

Epidemiologically, physical activity has been decreasing in the last decades [2], even more before the year of 2000, after which the trend stabilised with negligible changes [3] apart from COVID-19 epidemics, where cardiorespiratory fitness declined significantly [4, 5]. The decline in the last decades was more pronounced in children over the school-age years. Boys were usually more fit than girls [6]. Cardiorespiratory fitness was found to be higher in socially advantaged children [7].

Lower cardiorespiratory fitness is associated with low physical activity and increased fat mass. Increasing obesity in children is therefore strongly inversely associated with cardiorespiratory fitness and indicates reduced physical activity in the paediatric population in recent decades. Interestingly, fitness scores also decreased among lean children [8]. Association between low cardiorespiratory fitness and metabolic risk factors might therefore be only partially mediated through obesity [9]. Sedentary time also negatively affects cardiorespiratory fitness [10], which is independently linked to poor metabolic health [10]. Physical activity and sedentary time are clearly interrelated but a reciprocal relationship between them cannot be assumed [11]. Physical activity and training undoubtedly improve cardiovascular fitness with high-intensity interval training being more successful in enhancing cardiovascular fitness compared to moderate-intensity continuous training [12].

Cardiorespiratory fitness has been also associated with inflammatory biomarkers in children with a positive association with body fat. Similarly, the association between lifestyle behaviours, such as diet, physical activity and sedentary behaviour, and inflammation were found in the paediatric population [13].

Improved cardiorespiratory fitness was associated with the reduced inflammatory profile, independently of body composition and lifestyle behaviours [13]. Cardiorespiratory fitness and sports-related physical activity were also inversely associated with arterial stiffness in young adults [14].

Low cardiorespiratory fitness is strongly associated with the clustering of cardiovascular risk factors in children [15]. Evaluation and improvement of cardiorespiratory fitness in children with cardiovascular risk factors might be associated with improved health parameters in later life [1]. In this review, we present methods on how to evaluate cardiovascular fitness in children along with available data on cardiovascular fitness in children with some traditional and novel cardiovascular risk factors. Some specific strategies to improve cardiovascular fitness in children are also added.

2. Cardiorespiratory fitness in children: how to measure it?

Cardiorespiratory fitness was clearly associated with body mass index, fat mass, and metabolic syndrome development, however, other cardiovascular risk factors are not always convincing in the literature. Partly, this might be the result of the different evaluation of cardiovascular fitness in different studies [16]. The barriers to cardiovascular fitness assessment include the lack of standardisation in the test protocols, the health outcome being evaluated as well as the absence of evidence-based clinical cut points at these ages [17].

The most widely used indicator of cardiorespiratory fitness is the volume of oxygen that is consumed at maximal physical exertion (VO_{2max}), measured from the respiratory gas exchange by indirect calorimetry [18]. It can be objectively and accurately measured through laboratory tests such as progressive run or cycle, however, these protocols require sophisticated equipment (run/cycle ergometer tests with respiratory gas analysis), the availability of trained technicians, making these tests expensive and time-consuming. Alternatively, field tests are more appropriate for universal screening and include a 550-m timed run/walk or "Maximal Multistage 20-m Shuttle Run Test" [18]. The latter was identified as the most scalable and reliable field test, where VO_{2max} can be predicted by special equations [19, 20]. For a field test to be valid it is required to accurately and reliably measure what it claims to measure, however, field-based tests usually suffer from low relative validity when compared to VO_{2max} measurement and are producing conflicting results [18, 21]. Other similar screening tests are being developed, such as the 3-minute Kasch Pulse Recovery Test, where a reference range for the classification of cardiorespiratory fitness was developed on the basis of the age-specific percentile distribution of heart rate after exercise in 6- to 9- and 10- to 12-year-old children. The value of heart rate after exercise is considered an indicator of cardiorespiratory fitness [22].

Another obstacle in the cardiorespiratory fitness evaluation is the lack of age-specific cut-off points for increased cardiovascular risk. They were attempted to be set by a systematic review in children aged 8–19 years that determined that fitness levels below 42 and 35 mL/kg/min (VO_{2max} measurement) for boys and girls, respectively, should raise a red flag. These cut-points identify children and adolescents who may benefit from primary and secondary cardiovascular prevention programming [17]. Similarly, a study using a 20-m Shuttle Run Test with VO_{2max} prediction by estimation revealed cut-off points in 8- to 12-year-olds for obesity identified as 39 mL/kg/min and 41 mL/kg/min for girls and boys, respectively [23].

Recommendations for future research must include standardised measurements with standardised outcome assessments of cardiorespiratory fitness. For universal screening, a field test approach might be more appropriate, however, in children with cardiovascular risk, or suboptimal results in the field test, a more accurate approach might be more appropriate with cut-off points determined for gender and age.

3. Cardiorespiratory fitness in children with obesity

Children with obesity have lower cardiorespiratory fitness than normal-weight children [24], which is more pronounced in girls [25] and is commonly associated with reduced physical activity [26]. Body mass index also mediates the association between cardiorespiratory fitness and metabolic syndrome in schoolchildren. Higher levels of cardiorespiratory fitness are associated with lower cardiometabolic risk, particularly, when accompanied by weight reduction [27]. Lower cardiorespiratory fitness in children with obesity was associated with overall and abdominal fat mass, whereas both central and total obesity were lower in overweight and obese children with high cardiorespiratory fitness [28–30]. There is extensive evidence to support the fat-but-fit paradigm, which shows that cardiorespiratory fitness can counteract the adverse effects of obesity on cardiovascular risk factors. Unfit children with obesity had exaggerated systolic blood pressure at rest and during sympathetic activation, presumably coupled with higher cardiac output and cardiac oxygen demand [31]. Even from the molecular point of view, fit children with obesity or overweight had a distinct pattern of whole-blood gene expression [32]. Concerning the autonomic nervous system's role, greater parasympathetic cardiac activity was associated with higher levels of cardiorespiratory fitness in both girls and boys, while the sympathetic-vagal balance was negatively related to maximal oxygen uptake in girls [33].

Additionally, in obesity, low-grade chronic inflammation and homeostatic stress produced mainly in adipocytes can result in abnormal adipokine secretion, which could be involved in the pathogenesis of lowered cardiorespiratory fitness. The secretion of adipokines is also influenced by physical fitness. It has been demonstrated that in children with obesity, VO_{2max} can be predicted from haematological parameters, such as leptin and fibrinogen [34].

4. Cardiorespiratory fitness in children with other traditional cardiovascular risk

4.1 Cardiorespiratory fitness in children with hypertension

Obesity-related hypertension is a problem on the rise with obesity epidemics. Cardiorespiratory fitness was associated with total and central obesity as well as hypertension [35, 36]. Systolic and diastolic blood pressure showed curvilinear relation with cardiorespiratory fitness along with waist circumference and the sum of skinfolds [37]. However, regardless of obesity, cardiorespiratory fitness in children has been associated with other metabolic risk factors and future health. Teenagers with low cardiorespiratory fitness were more likely to develop hypertension in adulthood, even among participants with a normal body mass index [24]. Children who are fit and participate regularly in sports outside school hours are less likely to be hypertensive [38]. Long-term low levels of cardiorespiratory fitness exhibited the highest levels of systolic blood pressure [39]. The combination of a family history of hypertension and cardiorespiratory fitness also showed a clear association with the increased risk of hypertension [40]. Interestingly, some studies set a different perspective on cardiorespiratory fitness and hypertension, somehow contradicting the above-mentioned associations. In one of them, physical activity was not associated with systolic blood pressure independently of adiposity, but there was a small independent association only with diastolic blood pressure [41]. Another study demonstrated that adolescents with overweight or obesity have a higher prevalence of higher blood pressure, regardless of cardiorespiratory fitness, suggesting that maintaining a normal body mass index protects against less favourable blood pressure [42]. Anyway, a study published two decades ago demonstrated that the level of cardiorespiratory fitness did not seem to be an important correlate of blood pressure variation across age groups and gender in schoolchildren [43].

4.2 Cardiorespiratory fitness in children with dyslipidaemia

Abnormal lipid profile is commonly known as a cardiovascular risk factor, sometimes associated with obesity, but in children, it can be the consequence of genetic defect leading to familial hypercholesterolemia also in lean children [44]. However, specific studies regarding familial hypercholesterolemia and cardiorespiratory fitness are lacking in the paediatric population. Overall, evidence supports an inverse association between cardiorespiratory fitness and dyslipidaemia with expected improvements in high-density lipoprotein cholesterol with exercise, which is the most consistent finding. The findings regarding the effects of exercise training on other lipid components have been variable, with both positive and null results, but in general demonstrate a reduction of total cholesterol and triglycerides with exercise training [45, 46]. Future studies in the paediatric population are needed to clarify the association between cardiorespiratory fitness change and dyslipidaemia [45].

4.3 Cardiorespiratory fitness in children with diabetes mellitus type 1 or type 2

Lower cardiorespiratory fitness, strength, and higher central adiposity were also highly predictive of higher levels of insulin resistance in children and adolescents without diabetes mellitus [47], however, at least in part, are mediated through obesity [48]. Nevertheless, increased muscle strength and cardiorespiratory fitness were associated with decreased insulin resistance and improved β-cell function among young in population studies [49, 50]. Cardiorespiratory fitness and muscular fitness in children are not only important in childhood but it was proven that they were inversely associated with measures of fasting insulin, insulin resistance, and β-cell function in adulthood [51].

In children with already developed diabetes mellitus, cardiorespiratory fitness might play an even more pivotal role. Independently of obesity, there was a significant inverse relationship between cardiorespiratory fitness and lipid profile components and systolic blood pressure in children with poorly controlled type 1 diabetes mellitus, indicating a favourable effect of increased cardiorespiratory fitness [52]. Additionally, youth with diabetes mellitus type 1 who are physically active, tend to have lower glycated haemoglobin and reduced insulin needs. Also, activity in adolescents at-risk for diabetes mellitus type 2 improves various measures of metabolism and body composition [53]. In children with diabetes mellitus type 2, lower levels of cardiorespiratory fitness were observed mostly due to physical inactivity [54]. People with diabetes mellitus type 2 have reduced cardiorespiratory fitness compared to healthy controls, with an association to increased cardiovascular morbidity and mortality. The mechanisms of lower cardiorespiratory fitness in children with diabetes mellitus type 2 are multifaceted and involve interrelated defects in insulin action, mitochondrial dysfunction, skeletal muscle microvasculature, and cardiac dysfunction [55]. In youth with diabetes mellitus type 2, left ventricular size is clearly related to physical fitness, which might counteract adverse effects of poor glycaemic control and, at least according to the study, right ventricular function [56]. Regular physical activity is an important component in the management of both diabetes mellitus type 1 and type 2, as it has the potential to improve glycaemic control, delay cardiovascular complications, and increase overall well-being [57].

5. Cardiorespiratory fitness in children with novel cardiovascular risk

5.1 Cardiorespiratory fitness in children with chronic kidney disease

Children with chronic kidney disease have lower cardiorespiratory fitness due to various reasons, one of the most important is reduced physical activity and increased sedentary lifestyle mainly due to the renal replacement therapy requirements (e.g. haemodialysis) [58]. Additionally, chronic kidney disease is associated with anaemia, effects of chronic uraemia, and metabolic acidosis on the heart and skeletal muscle, all contributing significantly to reduce physical activity [59]. Paediatric patients with chronic kidney disease are therefore significantly physically inactive, with less than 10% of the non-school time being physically active [60]. Additionally, children after kidney transplantation significantly gained fat weight [60, 61]. One of the reasons after transplantation might also be related to sirolimus effects on skeletal muscle [61]. Reduced cardiorespiratory fitness was strongly associated with the clustering of cardiovascular risk factors in these children [62].

Studies suggest that regular and early implementation of both aerobic and resistance exercise programs in persons with chronic kidney disease have positive effects on muscle function, exercise tolerance, and quality of life [59]. In children with a successful renal transplant, a weekly physical exercise of 3–5 hours significantly improved cardiorespiratory fitness and left ventricular mass [63].

In children with a congenital single kidney, physical activity improved aerobic capacity and exercise tolerance without increasing the risks of cardiovascular accidents [64], however, in the patients contact sports might be discouraged due to the increased risk of sport-related injury.

5.2 Cardiorespiratory fitness in children born prematurely

Children and also later adults, born prematurely, are likely to have poorer cardiorespiratory fitness, however, according to some studies, the poor cardiorespiratory outcome of a child born prematurely is not firmly established [65, 66]. In adults, exercise capacity was only modestly reduced and frequently with values within a normal range and was consistent with self-reported exercise capacity [67]. In addition, in children with abnormal lung function and structure, this did not impact the aerobic exercise capacity of preterm children at school age [68]. On the contrary, Welsh et al. demonstrated a significant reduction in peak oxygen consumption among prematurely born children but with no difference in physical activity [69]. Some subgroups of premature-born individuals might be at increased risk for reduced cardiorespiratory fitness, especially those with lower muscular fitness, which was more common among premature-born young adults [70]. Lowered muscle strength is associated also with neuromotor sequelae of premature birth [71]. Another risk factor for reduced exercise capacity is also a decreased ventricular size and mass that might be a consequence of prematurity [72]. Impaired heart rate recovery after maximal exercise might also play a role in poor cardiorespiratory fitness in some suggesting an impaired development of autonomic nervous function after preterm labour [73].

Babies, born prematurely, are a diverse group of patients with complications that depend on several factors, such as gestational age, associated comorbidities, prenatal factors, postnatal care, etc. Therefore, the studies are diverse and might contradict each other because the effect of premature birth depends on so many other factors. Anyway, children born prematurely do have a risk for lowered cardiorespiratory fitness and regular physical intervention is believed to produce better outcomes [65, 71].

5.3 Cardiorespiratory fitness in children with congenital heart disease

Congenital heart disease may in a variety of ways adversely affect hemodynamic responses, usually produced during exercises, such as increased heart rate, preload, and heart contractility with decreased systemic vascular resistance and pulmonary vascular resistance [74]. Therefore, the consequences of cardiorespiratory fitness depend on the congenital defect itself and a proper evaluation is of pivotal importance to evaluate cardiac rehabilitation. Historically, children with congenital heart disease have been restricted from exercise, contributing to a sedentary lifestyle as well as increased cardiovascular risk factors. Given the large benefits and small risks of exercise in this population, guidelines have recently shifted towards exercise promotion [75]. In children, several tests to evaluate cardiorespiratory fitness might be used [74], however, the 6-minute walk test is quite common and was found to be a useful and reliable tool in the assessment and follow-up of functional capacity during rehabilitation programs [76]. Furthermore, exercise training is safe and beneficial for the vast majority of adults with congenital heart disease following appropriate screening [77, 78].

Exercise recommendations should be individualised based on functional parameters using a structured methodology to approach the evaluation, risk classification, and prescriptions of exercise and physical activity [75]. Participation in aerobic exercise significantly increased the quality of life in children with congenital heart disease [79].

6. Cardiorespiratory fitness, sleep and psychosocial well-being

Sleeping quality was also associated with cardiorespiratory fitness, not necessarily in children with high body mass index, as might be expected. Girls who were classified as fit were more likely to report better sleep quality compared to their unfit peers. Poor sleep quality was associated with lower cardiorespiratory fitness with no significant association with body mass index [80].

Not only obesity reduction, but improved cardiorespiratory fitness also positively affects psychosocial well-being, leading to improved self-esteem and reduced stress, further reducing cardiovascular risk. Cognitive function and cardiorespiratory fitness correlate significantly and are predictors of psychological well-being among school-aged children. In addition, students with a higher level of psychological well-being showed a higher cardiorespiratory fitness, concentration performance, and attention accuracy [81]. Cardiorespiratory fitness also had a small protective effect against developing depression [82]. Similarly, it was found that stress and depression can affect an individual's level of physical activity and fitness, which may place them at risk of developing cardiovascular disease, confirming the role of increased physical activity in improving depression and reducing depression-related stress to improve cardiovascular risk [83].

7. Strategies to improve cardiorespiratory fitness in children

Addressing cardiovascular fitness in children and adolescents could reduce future adiposity, improve other cardiovascular risk factors and thus be an important factor in improving health [16]. The main strategies for reducing cardiovascular risk and obesity remain physical exercise with a reduced sedentary lifestyle and an appropriate diet. Promoting health-related cardiorespiratory fitness in physical education proved to be an important contributor to improving cardiorespiratory fitness in children. Intensity, age, and weight status importantly affect cardiorespiratory fitness [84]. In children with obesity, regular exercise is even more important, and may not need to be vigorous; recreational programs are also effective and may encourage children to participate in physical activity and limit initial dropout. Three-month training programs in children with obesity led to decreased body mass index, waist circumference, decreased fat mass, blood glucose, homeostasis model assessment for insulin resistance, triglycerides, and systolic pressure before and after exercise [85].

A healthier diet in preschool and schoolchildren also led to lower adiposity levels, lower waist circumference, and increased cardiorespiratory fitness, making it a relevant modifiable factor in obesity management [86, 87].

The management of the whole family is of utmost importance because a parent's effect can have a significant impact on children's willingness and motivation to change their lifestyle [88]. Breastfeeding has also been positively associated with cardiorespiratory fitness, where breastfeeding for more than 6 months proved to have positive

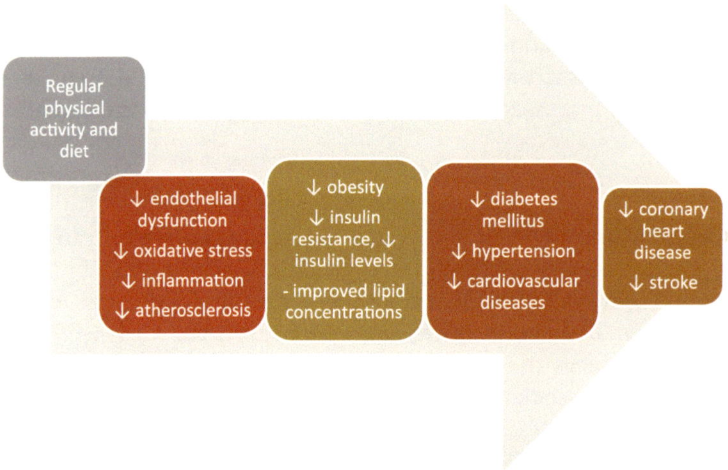

Figure 1.
From regular physical activity and diet to decreased morbidity and mortality due to the cardiovascular diseases.

effects on cardiorespiratory fitness. Therefore, early nutrition may be a predictor for adolescence physical health and is of special importance to promoting healthier lifestyle in children as it is associated with higher cardiorespiratory fitness [89].

Intervention strategies aiming to reduce obesity and improve cardiorespiratory fitness in childhood might contribute to the prevention of metabolic syndrome in adulthood [90]. The process is schematically presented in **Figure 1**.

8. Conclusions

Cardiorespiratory fitness is declining in the paediatric population and is closely associated with increased cardiovascular risk. In children already having a cardiovascular risk factor present, it is important to determine cardiorespiratory fitness and if it is decreased, prompt physical intervention is warranted. Further research is needed to establish a standardised protocol of its measurement. Interventions include increased and customized physical activity along with a healthy diet. In children, breastfeeding could present an additional preventive factor.

Conflict of interest

The authors declare no conflict of interest.

Author details

Mirjam Močnik[1*] and Nataša Marčun Varda[1,2]

1 Department of Paediatrics, University Medical Centre Maribor, Maribor, Slovenia

2 University Medical Centre Maribor and Medical Faculty, Department of Paediatrics, University of Maribor, Maribor, Slovenia

*Address all correspondence to: mirjammocnik91@gmail.com

References

[1] García-Hermoso A, Ramírez-Vélez R, García-Alonso Y, Alonso-Martínez AM, Izquierdo M. Association of cardiorespiratory fitness levels during youth with health risk later in life: A systematic review and meta-analysis. JAMA Pediatrics. 2020;**174**:952-960. DOI: 10.1001/jamapediatrics.2020.2400

[2] Eberhardt T, Niessner C, Oriwol D, Buchal L, Worth A, Bös K. Secular trends in physical fitness of children and adolescents: A review of large-scale epidemiological studies published after 2006. International Journal of Environmental Research and Public Health. 2020;**17**:5671. DOI: 10.3390/ijerph17165671

[3] Tomkinson GR, Lang JJ, Tremblay MS. Temporal trends in the cardiorespiratory fitness of children and adolescents representing 19 high-income and upper middle-income countries between 1981 and 2014. British Journal of Sports Medicine. 2019;**53**:478-486. DOI: 10.1136/bjsports-2017-097982

[4] Jarnig G, Jaunig J, van Poppel MNM. Association of COVID-19 mitigation measures with changes in cardiorespiratory fitness and body mass index among children aged 7 to 10 years in Austria. JAMA Network Open. 2021;**4**:e2121675. DOI: 10.1001/jamanetworkopen.2021.21675

[5] López-Bueno R, Calatayud J, Andersen LL, Casaña J, Ezzatvar Y, Casajús JA, et al. Cardiorespiratory fitness in adolescents before and after the COVID-19 confinement: A prospective cohort study. European Journal of Pediatrics. 2021;**180**:2287-2293. DOI: 10.1007/s00431-021-04029-8

[6] Sallis JF. Epidemiology of physical activity and fitness in children and adolescents. Critical Reviews in Food Science and Nutrition. 1993;**33**:403-408. DOI: 10.1080/10408399309527639

[7] Okely AD, Hardy LL, Booth ML, Dobbins TA, Denney-Wilson EA, Yang B. Changes in cardiorespiratory fitness among children and adolescents in Australia: 1997 and 2004. Journal of Sports Sciences. 2010;**28**:851-857. DOI: 10.1080/02640411003716959

[8] Stratton G, Canoy D, Boddy LM, Taylor SR, Hackett AF, Buchan IE. Cardiorespiratory fitness and body mass index of 9-11-year-old English children: A serial cross-sectional study from 1998 to 2004. International Journal of Obesity. 2007;**31**:1172-1178. DOI: 10.1038/sj.ijo.0803562

[9] Ekelund U, Anderssen SA, Froberg K, Sardinha LB, Andersen LB, Brage S, et al. Independent associations of physical activity and cardiorespiratory fitness with metabolic risk factors in children: The European youth heart study. Diabetologia. 2007;**50**:1832-1840. DOI: 10.1007/s00125-007-0762-5

[10] Moore JB, Beets MW, Barr-Anderson DJ, Evenson KR. Sedentary time and vigorous physical activity are independently associated with cardiorespiratory fitness in middle school youth. Journal of Sports Sciences. 2013;**31**:1520-1525. DOI: 10.1080/02640414.2013.793378

[11] Sandercock GR, Ogunleye AA. Independence of physical activity and screen time as predictors of cardiorespiratory fitness in youth. Pediatric Research. 2013;**73**:692-697. DOI: 10.1038/pr.2013.37

[12] Cao M, Quan M, Zhuang J. Effect of high-intensity interval training

versus moderate-intensity continuous training on cardiorespiratory fitness in children and adolescents: A meta-analysis. International Journal of Environmental Research and Public Health. 2019;**16**:1533. DOI: 10.3390/ijerph16091533

[13] González-Gil EM, Santaliestra-Pasías AM, Buck C, Gracia-Marco L, Lauria F, Pala V, et al. Improving cardiorespiratory fitness protects against inflammation in children: The IDEFICS study. Pediatric Research. 2022;**91**:681-689. DOI: 10.1038/s41390-021-01471-0

[14] Boreham CA, Ferreira I, Twisk JW, Gallagher AM, Savage MJ, Murray LJ. Cardiorespiratory fitness, physical activity, and arterial stiffness: The Northern Ireland Young Hearts Project. Hypertension. 2004;**44**:721-726. DOI: 10.1161/01.HYP.0000144293.40699.9a

[15] Anderssen SA, Cooper AR, Riddoch C, Sardinha LB, Harro M, Brage S, et al. Low cardiorespiratory fitness is a strong predictor for clustering of cardiovascular disease risk factors in children independent of country, age and sex. European Journal of Cardiovascular Prevention and Rehabilitation. 2007;**14**:526-531. DOI: 10.1097/HJR.0b013e328011efc1

[16] Mintjens S, Menting MD, Daams JG, van Poppel MNM, Roseboom TJ, Gemke RJBJ. Cardiorespiratory fitness in childhood and adolescence affects future cardiovascular risk factors: A systematic review of longitudinal studies. Sports Medicine. 2018;**48**:2577-2605. DOI: 10.1007/s40279-018-0974-5

[17] Ruiz JR, Cavero-Redondo I, Ortega FB, Welk GJ, Andersen LB, Martinez-Vizcaino V. Cardiorespiratory fitness cut points to avoid cardiovascular disease risk in children and adolescents; what level of fitness should raise a red flag? A systematic review and meta-analysis. British Journal of Sports Medicine. 2016;**50**:1451-1458. DOI: 10.1136/bjsports-2015-095903

[18] Hamlin MJ, Fraser M, Lizamore CA, Draper N, Shearman JP, Kimber NE. Measurement of cardiorespiratory fitness in children from two commonly used field tests after accounting for body fatness and maturity. Journal of Human Kinetics. 2014;**40**:83-92. DOI: 10.2478/hukin-2014-0010

[19] Domone S, Mann S, Sandercock G, Wade M, Beedie C. A method by which to assess the scalability of field-based fitness tests of cardiorespiratory fitness among schoolchildren. Sports Medicine. 2016;**46**:1819-1831. DOI: 10.1007/s40279-016-0553-6

[20] Léger LA, Mercier D, Gadoury C, Lambert J. The multistage 20 metre shuttle run test for aerobic fitness. Journal of Sports Sciences. 1988;**6**:93-101. DOI: 10.1080/02640418808729800

[21] Boreham CA, Paliczka VJ, Nichols AK. A comparison of the PWC170 and 20-MST tests of aerobic fitness in adolescent schoolchildren. The Journal of Sports Medicine and Physical Fitness 1990;**30**:19-23

[22] Jankowski M, Niedzielska A, Brzezinski M, Drabik J. Cardiorespiratory fitness in children: A simple screening test for population studies. Pediatric Cardiology. 2015;**36**:27-32. DOI: 10.1007/s00246-014-0960-0

[23] Silva DAS, Lang JJ, Barnes JD, Tomkinson GR, Tremblay MS. Cardiorespiratory fitness in children: Evidence for criterion-referenced cut-points. PLoS One. 2018;**13**:e0201048. DOI: 10.1371/journal.pone.0201048

[24] Johansson L, Brissman M, Morinder G, Westerståhl M, Marcus C. Reference values and secular trends for cardiorespiratory fitness in children and adolescents with obesity. Acta Paediatrica. 2020;**109**:1665-1671. DOI: 10.1111/apa.15163

[25] Mota J, Flores L, Flores L, Ribeiro JC, Santos MP. Relationship of single measures of cardiorespiratory fitness and obesity in young schoolchildren. American Journal of Human Biology. 2006;**18**:335-341. DOI: 10.1002/ajhb.20513

[26] Maggio AB, Hofer MF, Martin XE, Marchand LM, Beghetti M, Farpour-Lambert NJ. Reduced physical activity level and cardiorespiratory fitness in children with chronic diseases. European Journal of Pediatrics. 2010;**169**:1187-1193. DOI: 10.1007/s00431-010-1199-2

[27] Díez-Fernández A, Sánchez-López M, Mora-Rodríguez R, Notario-Pacheco B, Torrijos-Niño C, Martínez-Vizcaíno V. Obesity as a mediator of the influence of cardiorespiratory fitness on cardiometabolic risk: A mediation analysis. Diabetes Care. 2014;**37**:855-862. DOI: 10.2337/dc13-0416

[28] Nassis GP, Psarra G, Sidossis LS. Central and total adiposity are lower in overweight and obese children with high cardiorespiratory fitness. European Journal of Clinical Nutrition. 2005;**59**:137-141. DOI: 10.1038/sj.ejcn.1602061

[29] Stigman S, Rintala P, Kukkonen-Harjula K, Kujala U, Rinne M, Fogelholm M. Eight-year-old children with high cardiorespiratory fitness have lower overall and abdominal fatness. International Journal of Pediatric Obesity. 2009;**4**:98-105. DOI: 10.1080/17477160802221101

[30] Lee SJ, Arslanian SA. Cardiorespiratory fitness and abdominal adiposity in youth. European Journal of Clinical Nutrition. 2007;**61**:561-565. DOI: 10.1038/sj.ejcn.1602541

[31] Legantis CD, Nassis GP, Dipla K, Vrabas IS, Sidossis LS, Geladas ND. Role of cardiorespiratory fitness and obesity on hemodynamic responses in children. The Journal of Sports Medicine and Physical Fitness. 2012;**52**:311-318

[32] Plaza-Florido A, Altmäe S, Esteban FJ, Löf M, Radom-Aizik S, Ortega FB. Cardiorespiratory fitness in children with overweight/obesity: Insights into the molecular mechanisms. Scandinavian Journal of Medicine & Science in Sports. 2021;**31**:2083-2091. DOI: 10.1111/sms.14028

[33] da Silva DF, Bianchini JA, Antonini VD, Hermoso DA, Lopera CA, Pagan BG, et al. Parasympathetic cardiac activity is associated with cardiorespiratory fitness in overweight and obese adolescents. Pediatric Cardiology. 2014;**35**:684-690. DOI: 10.1007/s00246-013-0838-6

[34] Tsiroukidou K, Hatziagorou E, Grammatikopoulou MG, Vamvakis A, Kontouli K, Tzimos C, et al. Cardiorespiratory fitness predicted by fibrinogen and leptin concentrations in children with obesity and risk for diabetes: A cross-sectional study and a ROC curve analysis. Nutrients. 2021;**13**:674. DOI: 10.3390/nu13020674

[35] Burgos MS, Reuter CP, Burgos LT, Pohl HH, Pauli LT, Horta JA, et al. Comparison analysis of blood pressure, obesity, and cardio-respiratory fitness in schoolchildren. Arquivos Brasileiros de Cardiologia. 2010;**94**:788-793. DOI: 10.1590/s0066-782x2010005000046

[36] Ruiz JR, Ortega FB, Loit HM, Veidebaum T, Sjöström M. Body fat is associated with blood pressure in school-

aged girls with low cardiorespiratory fitness: The European Youth Heart Study. Journal of Hypertension. 2007;**25**:2027-2034. DOI: 10.1097/HJH.0b013e328277597f

[37] Klasson-Heggebø L, Andersen LB, Wennlöf AH, Sardinha LB, Harro M, Froberg K, et al. Graded associations between cardiorespiratory fitness, fatness, and blood pressure in children and adolescents. British Journal of Sports Medicine. 2006;**40**:25-29. DOI: 10.1136/bjsm.2004.016113

[38] Nqweniso S, Walter C, du Randt R, Aerts A, Adams L, Degen J, et al. Prevention of overweight and hypertension through cardiorespiratory fitness and extracurricular sport participation among South African schoolchildren. Sustainability. 2020;**12**:6581. DOI: 10.3390/su12166581

[39] Agostinis-Sobrinho C, Ruiz JR, Moreira C, Abreu S, Lopes L, Oliveira-Santos J, et al. Cardiorespiratory fitness and blood pressure: A longitudinal analysis. The Journal of Pediatrics. 2018;**192**:130-135. DOI: 10.1016/j.jpeds.2017.09.055

[40] Gando Y, Sawada SS, Kawakami R, Momma H, Shimada K, Fukunaka Y, et al. Combined association of cardiorespiratory fitness and family history of hypertension on the incidence of hypertension: A long-term cohort study of Japanese males. Hypertension Research. 2018;**41**:1063-1069. DOI: 10.1038/s41440-018-0117-2

[41] Hunt LP, Shield JP, Cooper AR, Ness AR, Lawlor DA. Blood pressure in children in relation to relative body fat composition and cardio-respiratory fitness. International Journal of Pediatric Obesity. 2011;**6**:275-284. DOI: 10.3109/17477166.2011.583655

[42] Bertollo C, Barbian CD, de Borba SL, de Castro Silveira JF, Vogt BD, de Mello ED, et al. Hypertension and different levels of body mass index and cardiorespiratory fitness amongst adolescents. International Journal of Cardiovascular Science. 2021;**36**(6):610-616. DOI: 10.36660/ijcs.20200038

[43] Guerra S, Ribeiro JC, Costa R, Duarte J, Mota J. Relationship between cardiorespiratory fitness, body composition and blood pressure in school children. The Journal of Sports Medicine and Physical Fitness. 2002;**42**:207-213

[44] Bogsrud MP, Langslet G, Wium C, Johansen D, Svilaas A, Holven KB. Treatment goal attainment in children with familial hypercholesterolemia: A cohort study of 302 children in Norway. Journal of Clinical Lipidology. 2018;**12**:375-382. DOI: 10.1016/j.jacl.2017.11.009

[45] Reuter CP, Brand C, Silva PTD, Reuter ÉM, Renner JDP, Franke SIR, Met al. Relationship between dyslipidemia, cultural factors, and cardiorespiratory fitness in schoolchildren. Arquivos Brasileiros de Cardiologia 2019;**112**:729-736. DOI: 10.5935/abc.20190068.

[46] Sui X, Sarzynski MA, Lee DC, Kokkinos PF. Impact of changes in cardiorespiratory fitness on hypertension, dyslipidemia and survival: An overview of the epidemiological evidence. Progress in Cardiovascular Diseases. 2017;**60**:56-66. DOI: 10.1016/j.pcad.2017.02.006

[47] Benson AC, Torode ME, Singh MA. Muscular strength and cardiorespiratory fitness is associated with higher insulin sensitivity in children and adolescents. International Journal of Pediatric Obesity. 2006;**1**:222-231. DOI: 10.1080/17477160600962864

[48] Lee S, Bacha F, Gungor N, Arslanian SA. Cardiorespiratory fitness

in youth: Relationship to insulin sensitivity and beta-cell function. Obesity (Silver Spring). 2006;**14**:1579-1585. DOI: 10.1038/oby.2006.182

[49] Grøntved A, Ried-Larsen M, Ekelund U, Froberg K, Brage S, Andersen LB. Independent and combined association of muscle strength and cardiorespiratory fitness in youth with insulin resistance and β-cell function in young adulthood: The European Youth Heart Study. Diabetes Care. 2013;**36**:2575-2581. DOI: 10.2337/dc12-2252

[50] Artero EG, Ruiz JR, Ortega FB, España-Romero V, Vicente-Rodríguez G, Molnar D, et al. Muscular and cardiorespiratory fitness are independently associated with metabolic risk in adolescents: The HELENA study. Pediatric Diabetes. 2011;**12**:704-712. DOI: 10.1111/j.1399-5448.2011.00769.x

[51] Fraser BJ, Blizzard L, Schmidt MD, Juonala M, Dwyer T, Venn AJ, et al. Childhood cardiorespiratory fitness, muscular fitness and adult measures of glucose homeostasis. Journal of Science and Medicine in Sport. 2018;**21**:935-940. DOI: 10.1016/j.jsams.2018.02.002

[52] Miculis CP, de Campos W, Gasparotto GS, Silva MP, Mascarenhas LP, Boguszewski MC. Correlation of cardiorespiratory fitness with risk factors for cardiovascular disease in children with type 1 diabetes mellitus. Journal of Diabetes and its Complications. 2012;**26**:419-423. DOI: 10.1016/j.jdiacomp.2012.05.011

[53] Pivovarov JA, Taplin CE, Riddell MC. Current perspectives on physical activity and exercise for youth with diabetes. Pediatric Diabetes. 2015;**16**:242-255. DOI: 10.1111/pedi.12272

[54] Shaibi GQ, Michaliszyn SB, Fritschi C, Quinn L, Faulkner MS. Type 2 diabetes in youth: A phenotype of poor cardiorespiratory fitness and low physical activity. International Journal of Pediatric Obesity. 2009;**4**:332-337. DOI: 10.3109/17477160902923341

[55] Abushamat LA, McClatchey PM, Scalzo RL, Schauer I, Huebschmann AG, Nadeau KJ, et al. Mechanistic causes of reduced cardiorespiratory fitness in type 2 diabetes. Journal of Endocrine Society. 2020;**4**:bvaa063. DOI: 10.1210/jendso/bvaa063

[56] Bacha F, Gidding SS, Pyle L, Levitt Katz L, Kriska A, Nadeau KJ, et al. Relationship of cardiac structure and function to cardiorespiratory fitness and lean body mass in adolescents and young adults with type 2 diabetes. The Journal of Pediatrics. 2016;**177**:159. DOI: 10.1016/j.jpeds.2016.06.048

[57] Nadella S, Indyk JA, Kamboj MK. Management of diabetes mellitus in children and adolescents: Engaging in physical activity. Translation Pediatrics. 2017;**6**:215-224. DOI: 10.21037/tp.2017.05.01

[58] Clark SL, Denburg MR, Furth SL. Physical activity and screen time in adolescents in the chronic kidney disease in children (CKiD) cohort. Pediatric Nephrology. 2016;**31**:801-808. DOI: 10.1007/s00467-015-3287-z

[59] Patel DR, Raj VM, Torres A. Chronic kidney disease, exercise, and sports in children, adolescents, and adults. The Physician and Sportsmedicine. 2009;**37**:11-19. DOI: 10.3810/psm.2009.10.1724

[60] Painter P, Krasnoff J, Mathias R. Exercise capacity and physical fitness in pediatric dialysis and kidney transplant patients. Pediatric Nephrology.

2007;**22**:1030-1039. DOI: 10.1007/s00467-007-0458-6

[61] Sethna CB, Salerno AE, McBride MG, Shults J, Paridon SM, Sharma N, et al. Cardiorespiratory fitness in pediatric renal transplant recipients. Transplantation. 2009;**88**:395-401. DOI: 10.1097/TP.0b013e3181aed7d1

[62] Tangeraas T, Midtvedt K, Fredriksen PM, Cvancarova M, Mørkrid L, Bjerre A. Cardiorespiratory fitness is a marker of cardiovascular health in renal transplanted children. Pediatric Nephrology. 2010;**25**:2343-2350. DOI: 10.1007/s00467-010-1596-9

[63] Lubrano R, Tancredi G, Bellelli E, Gentile I, Scateni S, Masciangelo R, et al. Influence of physical activity on cardiorespiratory fitness in children after renal transplantation. Nephrology, Dialysis, Transplantation. 2012;**27**:1677-1681. DOI: 10.1093/ndt/gfr434

[64] Tancredi G, Lambiase C, Favoriti A, Ricupito F, Paoli S, Duse M, et al. Cardiorespiratory fitness and sports activities in children and adolescents with solitary functioning kidney. Italian Journal of Pediatrics. 2016;**42**:43. DOI: 10.1186/s13052-016-0255-6

[65] Ferreira I, Gbatu PT, Boreham CA. Gestational age and cardiorespiratory fitness in individuals born at term: A life course study. Journal of the American Heart Association. 2017;**6**:e006467. DOI: 10.1161/JAHA.117.006467

[66] Kosiecz A, Chrościńska-Krawczyk M, Taczała J, Zawadka M. Evaluation of physical and cardiorespiratory fitness in 7-year-old prematurely born children – preliminary study. Annals of Agricultural and Environmental Medicine. 2021;**28**:502-508. DOI: 10.26444/aaem/127220

[67] Clemm HH, Vollsæter M, Røksund OD, Eide GE, Markestad T, Halvorsen T. Exercise capacity after extremely preterm birth. Development from adolescence to adulthood. Annals of the American Thoracic Society. 2014;**11**:537-545. DOI: 10.1513/AnnalsATS.201309-311OC

[68] O'Dea CA, Logie K, Wilson AC, Pillow JJ, Murray C, Banton G, et al. Lung abnormalities do not influence aerobic capacity in school children born preterm. European Journal of Applied Physiology. 2021;**121**:489-498. DOI: 10.1007/s00421-020-04530-2

[69] Welsh L, Kirkby J, Lum S, Odendaal D, Marlow N, Derrick G, et al. The EPICure study: Maximal exercise and physical activity in school children born extremely preterm. Thorax. 2010;**65**:165-172. DOI: 10.1136/thx.2008.107474

[70] Tikanmäki M, Tammelin T, Sipola-Leppänen M, Kaseva N, Matinolli HM, Miettola S, et al. Physical fitness in young adults born preterm. Pediatrics. 2016;**137**(1):e20151289. DOI: 10.1542/peds.2015-1289

[71] Lowe J, Cousins M, Kotecha SJ, Kotecha S. Physical activity outcomes following preterm birth. Paediatric Respiratory Reviews. 2017;**22**:76-82. DOI: 10.1016/j.prrv.2016.08.012

[72] McKay L, Goss KN, Haraldsdottir K, Beshish AG, Barton GP, Palta M, et al. Decreased ventricular size and mass mediate the reduced exercise capacity in adolescents and adults born premature. Early Human Development. 2021;**160**:105426. DOI: 10.1016/j.earlhumdev.2021.105426

[73] Haraldsdottir K, Watson AM, Beshish AG, Pegelow DF, Palta M, Tetri LH, et al. Heart rate recovery

after maximal exercise is impaired in healthy young adults born preterm. European Journal of Applied Physiology. 2019;**119**:857-866. DOI: 10.1007/s00421-019-04075-z

[74] Rhodes J, Ubeda Tikkanen A, Jenkins KJ. Exercise testing and training in children with congenital heart disease. Circulation. 2010;**122**:1957-1967. DOI: 10.1161/CIRCULATIONAHA.110.958025

[75] Hansen K, Tierney S. Every child with congenital heart disease should be exercising. Current Opinion in Cardiology. 2022;**37**:91-98. DOI: 10.1097/HCO.0000000000000931

[76] Moalla W, Gauthier R, Maingourd Y, Ahmaidi S. Six-minute walking test to assess exercise tolerance and cardiorespiratory responses during training program in children with congenital heart disease. International Journal of Sports Medicine. 2005;**26**:756-762. DOI: 10.1055/s-2004-830558

[77] Tran D, Maiorana A, Ayer J, Lubans DR, Davis GM, Celermajer DS, et al. Recommendations for exercise in adolescents and adults with congenital heart disease. Progress in Cardiovascular Diseases. 2020;**63**:350-366. DOI: 10.1016/j.pcad.2020.03.002

[78] Thaulow E, Fredriksen PM. Exercise and training in adults with congenital heart disease. International Journal of Cardiology. 2004;**97**(Suppl. 1):35-38. DOI: 10.1016/j.ijcard.2004.08.007

[79] Dulfer K, Duppen N, Kuipers IM, Schokking M, van Domburg RT, Verhulst FC, et al. Aerobic exercise influences quality of life of children and youngsters with congenital heart disease: A randomized controlled trial. The Journal of Adolescent Health. 2014;**55**:65-72. DOI: 10.1016/j.jadohealth.2013.12.010

[80] Mota J, Vale S. Associations between sleep quality with cardiorespiratory fitness and BMI among adolescent girls. American Journal of Human Biology. 2010;**22**:473-475. DOI: 10.1002/ajhb.21019

[81] Chen W, Gu X, Chen J, Wang X. Association of cardiorespiratory fitness and cognitive function with psychological well-being in school-aged children. International Journal of Environmental Research and Public Health. 2022;**19**:1434. DOI: 10.3390/ijerph19031434

[82] Ruggero CJ, Petrie T, Sheinbein S, Greenleaf C, Martin S. Cardiorespiratory fitness may help in protecting against depression among middle school adolescents. The Journal of Adolescent Health. 2015;**57**:60-65. DOI: 10.1016/j.jadohealth.2015.03.016

[83] Olive LS, Telford RM, Byrne DG, Abhayaratna WP, Telford RD. Psychological distress leads to reduced physical activity and fitness in children: The Australian longitudinal LOOK study. Journal of Behavioral Medicine. 2016;**39**:587-598. DOI: 10.1007/s10865-016-9723-0

[84] Peralta M, Henriques-Neto D, Gouveia ÉR, Sardinha LB, Marques A. Promotinghealth-relatedcardiorespiratory fitness in physical education: A systematic review. PLoS One. 2020;**15**:e0237019. DOI: 10.1371/journal.pone.0237019

[85] Calcaterra V, Larizza D, Codrons E, De Silvestri A, Brambilla P, Abela S, et al. Improved metabolic and cardiorespiratory fitness during a recreational training program in obese children. Journal of Pediatric Endocrinology & Metabolism. 2013;**26**:271-276. DOI: 10.1515/jpem-2012-0157

[86] Labayen Goñi I, Arenaza L, Medrano M, García N, Cadenas-

Sanchez C, Ortega FB. Associations between the adherence to the Mediterranean diet and cardiorespiratory fitness with total and central obesity in preschool children: The PREFIT project. European Journal of Nutrition. 2018;**57**:2975-2983. DOI: 10.1007/s00394-017-1571-3

[87] Tambalis KD, Panagiotakos DB, Psarra G, Sidossis LS. Association of cardiorespiratory fitness levels with dietary habits and lifestyle factors in schoolchildren. Applied Physiology, Nutrition, and Metabolism. 2019;**44**:539-545. DOI: 10.1139/apnm-2018-0407

[88] Parekh N, Henriksson P, Delisle Nyström C, Silfvernagel K, Ruiz JR, Ortega FB, et al. Associations of parental self-efficacy with diet, physical activity, body composition, and cardiorespiratory fitness in Swedish preschoolers: Results from the MINISTOP Trial. Health Education & Behavior. 2018;**45**:238-246. DOI: 10.1177/1090198117714019

[89] Vafa M, Heshmati J, Sadeghi H, Shidfar F, Namazi N, Baradaran H, et al. Is exclusive breastfeeding and its duration related to cardiorespiratory fitness in childhood? The Journal of Maternal-Fetal & Neonatal Medicine. 2016;**29**:461-465. DOI: 10.3109/14767058.2015.1004052

[90] Christodoulos AD, Douda HT, Tokmakidis SP. Cardiorespiratory fitness, metabolic risk, and inflammation in children. International Journal of Pediatrics. 2012;**2012**:270515. DOI: 10.1155/2012/270515

Chapter 7

Effect of Hypertension on ECG Parameters

Abirlal Sen and Geeta Baruah

Abstract

Introduction: Across the world the prevalence of hypertension and other cardiovascular diseases are increasing at an alarming rate. These diseases also affect the young age and medical students are no exception. In this study, ECG variables like R-R interval, QRS Axis of the medical students along with their Blood pressure were recorded and the relationship between ECG variables and Blood pressure was studied. Materials and methods: The study was done in Dept. of Physiology, Jorhat Medical College. Sample size was calculated as 160 using EpiTools Software. Recording of Electrocardiogram and Blood pressure of 160 students were done. P values were calculated by Anova test in case of > two variables. Tukey HSD test was used for Post hoc analysis. Scatter diagrams were used to see relationship between study variables. P value <0.05 was considered as significant. Results: Comparison of ECG Variables between hypotensive, normotensive and hypertensive students showed that R-R Interval decreased significantly from 21.37 ± 4.24 in hypotensives to 19.74 ± 3.39 in normotensives and 18.27 ± 4.07 in hypertensive students. QRS Axis decreased from 75.35 ± 10.99 degrees in hypotensives to 54.80 ± 34.94 degrees in normotensives and 50.43 ± 25.59 degrees in hypertensive students. Conclusion: Changing of life style that includes reduced consumption of fat rich diets, fast foods, red meat and salt, performing regular physical exercises, and regular health check up in the form of Blood pressure and Electrocardiogram recording could be beneficial for the students to identify and take preventive measures against any cardiovascular ailments..

Keywords: medical students, heart rate, R-R interval, QRS Axis, blood pressure, hypertension

1. Introduction

Across the world the prevalence of non communicable diseases are increasing at an alarming rate. Among them hypertension and other cardiovascular diseases are common.

Cardiovascular disease (CVD) is a major cause of disability and premature death throughout the world. There are obvious signs of cardiovascular diseases that can be seen long before they occur [1]. The fatal complications of CVD are usually seen in middle-aged or elderly people. However, the pathological processes begins early in life and progresses gradually through adolescence and early adulthood. Thus, these cardiovascular diseases also affect the younger generation and medical students are no exception.

In cardiac medicine, resting electrocardiography (ECG) has proved its value as a diagnostic tool for detecting "silent" heart disease [2, 3]. Apart from its use in the clinical field, the ECG has also been employed as a prognostic tool in relatively healthy subjects. Therefore, accurate estimation of the true prevalence of ECG abnormalities in large samples helps in interpretation of the predictive value of ECG findings [4].

So to make the medical students aware and to sort out the risk factors affecting cardiac health, resting ECG is done as it serves as a better guide for risk-reduction therapies [5].

There is also growing incidence of hypertension occurring in younger ages as compared to older age groups in the past. It affects nearly a quarter of the adult population worldwide [6].Hypertension is an independent predictor of cardiovascular diseaseas. Such studies were done among young students in other parts of the world [7].

1.1 Purpose of the study

Medical students being the future physicians must be aware of their own health. In the present study an attempt has been made to assess Electrocardiographic parameters (R-RInterval, QRS Axis) and Blood pressure (BP) of medical students and to find the relationship between them.

2. Materials and methods

The present study was done in Dept. of Physiology, Jorhat Medical College. It was an institution based cross-sectional observational study. Study population included undergraduate medical students of Jorhat Medical College. Sampling technique used was simple random sampling. Considering prevalence of obesity as 24% [8] and 11% as desired precision under 95% confidence interval, sample size was calculated and rounded up to 160 using EpiTools Software.

The study included student volunteers of age 17–25 years who were non-smokers and gave consent for the study. The study excluded those students who did not take part in all the test procedures required for the study. Ethical Clearance was obtained from Institutional Ethical Committee (H), Jorhat Medical College, Jorhat.

2.1 Procedure of recording electrocardiogram

The Model BPL CARDIART 108 T-DIGI with single channel ECG recorder was used. The recordings were carried out according to the specifications of the American Heart Association, i.e. subjects lying supine with arms on sides, limb electrodes on the wrists and ankles, recording done at 25 mm/sec and calibrated at 10 mm/mV.

Informed written Consent was taken from the students. For the female students, the ECGs were conducted with the help of a female Lab attendant. The name of the subject with date and time of the recording was put on the recorded graph and the ECG jelly was removed using cotton. Heart rate (R-R Interval), QRS duration, frontal plane QRS axis from the ECGs were evaluated and then entered in computer and stored for further analysis.

2.1.1 Standardisations of ECG measurements

Were done everyday in the morning around 11 am on the dates of recording the Electrocardiogram.

2.2 Measurement of blood pressure (BP)

Littman 3 M Classic stethoscope was used. Diamond BPMR 120 Conventional Mercurial Type BP Machine was used. BP was recorded in a quiet, warm setting. The subject was asked to sit quietly with the back supported for five minutes and the arm supported at the level of heart. The subject was advised not to take any caffeine or exogenous adrenergic stimulants during the hour preceding the recording.

Before recording the blood pressure, it was ensured that the upper meniscus of the mercury coincided with the 'zero' of the mercury manometer. The BP was taken with subject's out-stretched right upper limb over the brachial artery, applying a cuff just above cubital fossa, using a mercury sphygmomanometer kept at level of subjects' heart in sitting position. Systolic blood pressure was first recorded by palpatory method and then systolic and diastolic blood pressure were recorded by auscultatory method. Categories of BP Used were as per American Heart Association 2017 Hypertension Guidelines [9].

2.3 Statistical analysis

The response frequencies and descriptive statistics like mean and standard deviation were calculated and analyzed by using MS Excel. P values were calculated using Anova Test by Interactive statistics software. Post-Hoc value comparison among the variables was done by using Tukey HSD Post hoc test. Scatter Diagrams were used to see the relationship between Study Variables. P value <0.05 was considered as significant.

3. Results

Distribution of Blood Pressure profile among 160 participants showed that, 119 students (74.38%) were normotensive, 33 students (20.62%) were hypertensive & 8 students (5%) were hypotensive (**Figure 1**).

Comparison of ECG Variables between hypotensive, normotensive and hypertensive students showed that R-R Interval decreased from 21.37 ± 4.24 in hypotensives to 19.74 ± 3.39 in normotensives and 18.27 ± 4.07 in hypertensive students. This finding came to be significant by Anova (p value 0.0393) (**Table 1**).

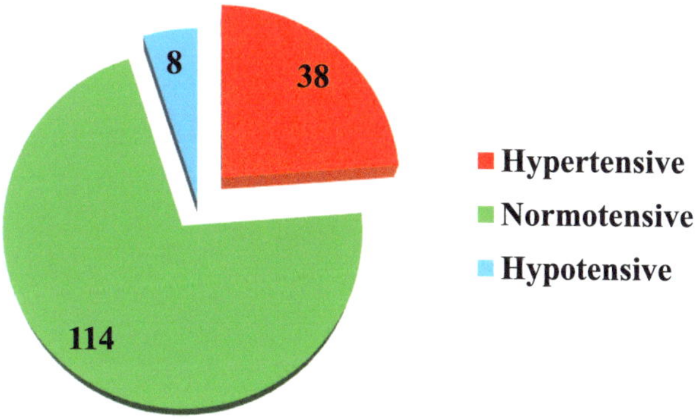

Figure 1.
Distribution of normotensives, hypertensives and hypotensives among the participants.

Parameters (Mean ± sd)	Hypotensives (n = 8)	Normotensives (n = 119)	Hypertensives (n = 33)	P value
R-R Interval	21.37 ± 4.24	19.74 ± 3.39	18.27 ± 4.07	0.0393*
QRS Axis (degrees)	75.35 ± 10.99	54.80 ± 34.94	50.43 ± 25.59	0.1536
Heart rate(beats/min)	73.01 ± 15.00	78.12 ± 12.89	85.69 ± 16.49	0.0095*

**statistically significant.*

Table 1.
Comparison of ECG variables between hypotensives, normotensives and hypertensives.

QRS Axis decreased from 75.35 ± 10.99 degrees in hypotensives to 54.80 ± 34.94 degrees in normotensives and 50.43 ± 25.59 degrees in hypertensive students. However, this finding was found to be insignificant by Anova (p value 0.1536). Heart rate increased from 73.01 ± 15.00 beats/min in hypotensives to 78.12 ± 12.89 beats/min in normotensives and 85.69 ± 16.49 beats/min in hypertensives. This comparison was found to be significant by Anova. (p value 0.0095) (**Table 1**).

By ANOVA test in **Table 1**, only the R-R interval,Heart rate differences between hypotensives, normotensives and hypertensives were found to be significant. (p value<0.05). After that, Tukey HSD Post-hoc Test revealed that among these Electrocacardiograhic parameters, only the Heart rate differences between the Normotensives and Hypertensives was found to be significant by Post-hoc analysis (p value =0.0163) in **Table 2**.

We found negative linear relationship of QRS Axis with Systolic BP i.e. as Systolic BP increased, QRS axis shifted toward left (**Figure 2**).

Negative linear relationship of QRS Axis with Diastolic BP i.e. as Diastolic BP increased, QRS axis shifted toward left (**Figure 3**).

A	
Parameters	**Post hoc p value of hypotensives(n = 8) vs. normotensives(n = 119)**
R-R Interval	0.4276
Heart rate	0.5691
B	
Parameters	**Post hoc p value of hypotensives(n = 8) vs hypertensives(n = 33)**
R-R Interval	0.0747
Heart rate	0.0543
C	
Parameters	**Post hoc p value of normotensives(n = 119) vs hypertensives(n = 33)**
R-R Interval	0.0957
Heart rate	**0.0163***

**Tukey HSD Post hoc significant.*

Table 2.
Post-hoc value comparison of the ECG variables between hypotensives, normotensives and hypertensives.

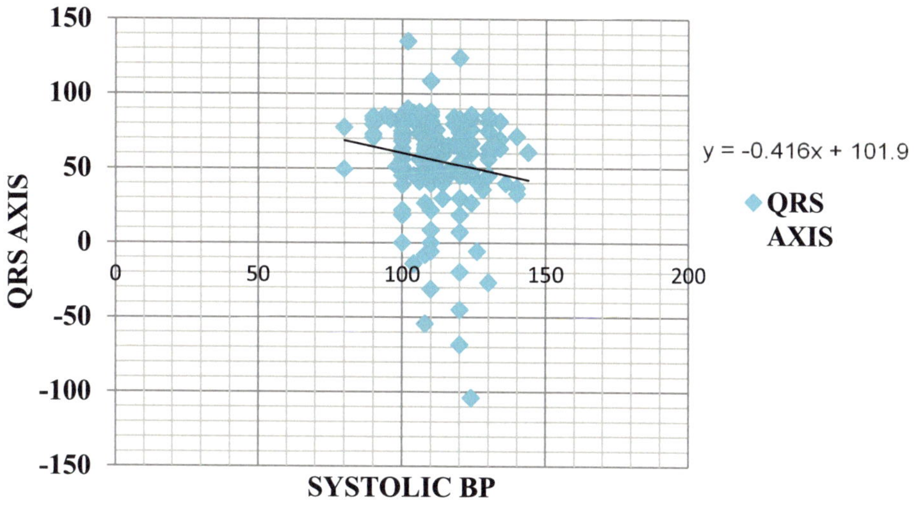

Figure 2.
Scatter diagram showing relationship of QRS Axis with systolic BP.

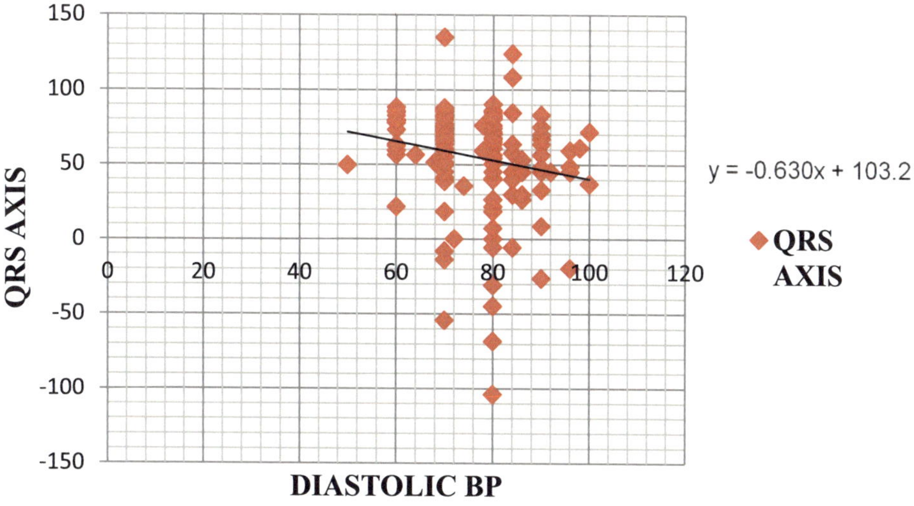

Figure 3.
Scatter diagram showing relationship of QRS Axis with diastolic BP.

4. Discussion

Our Study found that with increase in blood pressure, there is decrease in R-R Interval i.e. there is increase in Heart rate as BP increases. This finding came to be significant by Anova test. Our study also found that with increase in both SBP and DBP, there is leftward shift of QRS Axis.

This was similar to the findings of Kuroda Kenje et al. [10] and Alpert et al. [5]. The latter study found similar results in normotensive obese patients (>twice the ideal weight) compared to healthy normotensive subjects [5].

The physiological basis can be explained by the fact that when one ventricle is hypertrophied,the axis of the heart shifts toward the hypertrophied ventricle. This is because greater quantity of muscle exists on the hypertrophied side of the heart than on the other side. So, greater electrical potential is generated on that side. Secondly, more time is required for the depolarization wave to travel through the hypertrophied ventricle than through the normal ventricle. So, the normal ventricle becomes depolarized first, then the hypertrophied ventricle, and this causes a strong vector from the normal side of the heart toward the hypertrophied side [11].

Hypertension (high arterial blood pressure), causes the left ventricle to hypertrophy to pump blood against elevated systemic arterial pressure. Thus, in this case, left axis deviation occurs [11].

India has an increasing trend of hypertension especially among the urban population due to economic development and modernization with changing lifestyle factors [12]. Sedentary life style, intake of calorie rich junk foods and automated working profile has made the environment conducive for high prevalence of non communicable diseases (NCDs).

The rate of progression of disease is influenced by cardiovascular risk factors like unhealthy diet, tobacco use, physical inactivity (which together result in obesity) and elevated blood pressure (hypertension). Continued exposure to these risk factors leads to further progression of the diseases, resulting gradually in atherosclerosis, narrowing of blood vessels and obstruction of blood flow to vital organs, such as the heart and the brain leading to mortality [13]. The socioeconomic development has changed the dietary intake, food consumption patterns, and physical activity levels over the years contributing to the problem of increasing cardiovascular diseases among the population [14].

4.1 Study limitations

This study was a Cross sectional study; as such the casual relationship of the risk factors could not be established. The data collection could not be generalized as it was was limited to students from a single institution.

Another limitation of the study was that our study was limited only to R-R Interval (Heart rate) and QRS Axis and did not include other ECG parameters. A single BP recording was taken because of time constraints as students had to go for their classes and clinical postings. Furthermore, it remained to be investigated whether left shift of QRS axis in the hypertensives was based on increased LVH because detailed echocardiographic assessments were lacking which leaves scope for further study.

5. Conclusion

Our study showed that increase in blood pressure is associated with increase in heart rate and leftward shift of QRS axis. We recommended for changing life style that includes reduced consumption of fat rich diets, fast foods, salt restriction, performing regular physical exercises, yoga, meditation, sticking to a routine time table for sports, study and sleeping hours.

Regular health check up in the form of blood pressure measurement, recording of Electrocardiogram could be beneficial for the students to prevent hypertension, cardiovascular diseases and the risk factors associated with it.

It is highly desirable for such studies to be initiated so as to tackle the burden of noncommunicable diseases among thenew-generation physicians.

Author details

Abirlal Sen[1*] and Geeta Baruah[2]

1 Department of Physiology, Tripura Medical College and Dr. BRAM Teaching Hospital, Tripura, India

2 Department of Physiology, Jorhat Medical College, Assam, India

*Address all correspondence to: drabirlalsen@gmail.com

References

[1] Eisenstein I, Edelstein J, Sarma R, Sanmarco M, Selvester RH. The electrocardiogram in obesity. Journal of Electrocardiology. 1982;**15**(2):115-118

[2] Fye WB. A history of the origin, evolution, and impact of electrocardiography. The American Journal of Cardiology. 1994;**73**(13):937-949

[3] Sox HC Jr, Garber AM, Littenberg B. The resting electrocardiogram as a screening test: A clinical analysis. Annals of Internal Medicine 1989;**111**(6):489-502

[4] Blackburn H, Keys A, Simonson E, Rautaharju P, Punsar S. The electrocardiogram in population studies: A classification system. Circulation. 1960;**21**(6):1160-1175

[5] Alpert MA, Terry BE, Cohen MV, Fan TM, Painter JA, Massey CV. The electrocardiogram in morbid obesity. The American Journal of Cardiology. 2000;**85**(7):908-910

[6] Sinha DL. Prehypertension, heart rate, obesity and their co-relation; survey on medical students. Gujarat Medical Journal. 2015;**70**(2)

[7] Erikssen G, Bodegard J, Bjørnholt JV, Liestøl K, Thelle DS, Erikssen J. Exercise testing of healthy men in a new perspective: From diagnosis to prognosis. European Heart Journal. 2004;**25**(11):978-986

[8] Satyanarayana P, Roy M, Parma C, Mounika V, Ravuri S, Manaswi C, et al. Assessment of lung functions in obese young adolescent medical students. Journal of Dental Medicine Science. 2014;**13**:17-20

[9] Whelton PK, Carey RM, Aronow WS, Casey DE, Collins KJ, Himmelfarb CD, et al. 2017 ACC/AHA/AAPA/ABC/ACPM/AGS/APhA/ASH/ASPC/NMA/PCNA guideline for the prevention, detection, evaluation, and management of high blood pressure in adults: A report of the American College of Cardiology/American Heart Association task force on clinical practice guidelines. Journal of the American College of Cardiology. 2018;**71**(19):e127-e248

[10] Kuroda K, Ogawa T, Kojima S, Wakimoto T, Seki A, Fujii M. Relationship between exercise-induced QRS Axis shift and multiple risk factors for coronary heart disease. Ningen Dock. 2012;**26**(6):945-950

[11] Hall JE, AC G. Guyton and Hall textbook of medical physiology. 13th Edition

[12] Gupta R. Trends in hypertension epidemiology in India. Journal of Human Hypertension. 2004;**18**(2):73-78

[13] World Health Organization. Prevention of Cardiovascular Disease. World Health Organization; 2007

[14] Mungreiphy NK, Kapoor S, Sinha R. Association between BMI, blood pressure, and age: Study among Tangkhul Naga tribal males of Northeast India. Journal of Anthropology. 2011;**2011**

Chapter 8

Diabetes – A Silent Killer: A Threat for Cardiorespiratory Fitness

Theyamma Joseph and Jacquline C. Vadasseril

Abstract

Type 2 Diabetes Mellitus (T2DM) is a noncommunicable, lifestyle-related chronic metabolic disorder of global involvement, characterized by elevated blood sugar levels, manifested by hyperglycaemia, polyuria, polydipsia and polyphagia. DM is associated with acute and chronic complications which lead to reduced quality of life, premature morbidity and mortality. T2DM is linked with overweight, obesity, reduced physical activity and a genetic component. T2DM is named a silent killer because the primary disease is silent at the early stage and usually gets diagnosed when presenting with a vascular event such as stroke or heart attack. Impaired cardiorespiratory fitness plays a crucial role in acceleration of cardiovascular complications resulting in premature organ damage, morbidity and mortality. Regular physical activity, resistance training and reduction in sedentary life style along with diet control and drugs help to control DM and prevent or delay complications. This chapter deals with diabetes as a disease, its prevalence, risk factors, signs and symptoms, pathophysiology, pathogenesis and underlying mechanisms, acute and chronic complications, along with measures to enhance cardiorespiratory fitness and control DM and a word of caution to the younger generation to be aware of the silent killer.

Keywords: risk factors, pathophysiology, complications, control, prevention, cardiorespiratory fitness, T2DM

1. Introduction

Diabetes Mellitus (DM) is a chronic, metabolic disease characterized by chronically elevated circulating blood glucose levels (hyperglycaemia, FBS>126 mg%) which occurs when the body becomes resistant to insulin or doesn't make enough insulin. There are two types of diabetes: Type 1 Diabetes Mellitus (T1DM) and Type 2 Diabetes Mellitus (T2DM). Type 1 DM usually begins in youth and is an autoimmune disorder resulting in complete destruction of pancreatic beta cells, and thereby no insulin is produced. The person has to depend on external insulin supply lifelong. T2DM accounts for 95% of cases seen in adults, characterized by insulin resistance, where the response to insulin in the muscles, liver and fat cells is inadequate. This condition is amenable to exercise and diet to enhance insulin sensitivity. Insulin is essential for muscle, liver and adipose tissue cells to store glucose. Insulin resistance and insulin deficiency lead to hyperglycaemia or increased levels of circulating blood glucose which can damage the blood vessels and nerve. As a result, serious damage can happen to the heart, blood vessels, eyes, kidneys and nerves [1, 2]. Type 2 DM was once considered as a disease of the economically affluent 'western countries' that occurred by middle age, but today, it is increasingly seen affecting the younger generation. Diabetes damages the large and small blood vessels resulting in end organ damage. Uncontrolled diabetes leads to increased risk of vascular disease caused by macrovascular (cardiovascular (CV), cerebrovascular and peripheral artery disease) and microvascular (diabetic retinopathy, nephropathy and neuropathy) complications [3]. Long-term complications of this noncommunicable, chronic lifestyle disease are a leading cause of end stage renal failure, adult-onset blindness and non-traumatic amputations. Diabetes leads to atherosclerotic cardiovascular disease, a major cause of disability, reduced quality of life, morbidity, mortality and premature death [4]. Treatment of diabetic complications often is more expensive and disheartening than diabetes itself. The burden of DM is often unaffordable to the common man in a developing country where free medical service is unavailable to all citizens.

2. Prevalence of diabetes mellitus

According to WHO, noncommunicable disease accounts for 74% of death globally. The global prevalence of DM increased from 108 million in 1980 to 422 million in 2019 and accounted for 1.6 million deaths and the ninth leading cause of global mortality. By 2035, nearly 592 million people are predicted to die of diabetes [5]. In developing countries, undiagnosed diabetes accounts for more than 50%, which means 231.9 million (one in two) adults are with undiagnosed diabetes worldwide. An urgent need for diabetes screening, treatment and preventive initiatives along with population education exists worldwide.

At national level, India stands second to China in the global diabetic population with 77 million people with diabetes. About 57% (43.9 million) of adults having diabetes are undiagnosed in India. Besides, 25.2 million adults are assessed to have Impaired Glucose Tolerance (IGT), and that is expected to reach 35.7 million by the year 2045 [6]. An estimated number of diabetes patients in the 20–79 age group was 74.2 million in 2021 and is likely to increase to 124.8 million in 2045 [7]. In 2019, India was reported to have 77 million cases of diabetes and 54% cases of undiagnosed diabetes with the cases of DM projected to reach 134 million by the year 2045 if unchecked.

According to an ICMR study, India DIABetes, prevalence of diabetes has increased from 3.5 to 8.7% in rural and from 5.8 to 15.5% in urban areas, and the prevalence of prediabetes was reported as 5.8–14.7% in rural to 7.2–16.2% in urban areas. The number of cases of prediabetes exceeds that of diabetes and will become full-blown diabetes in a short span of 10 years. This will have a detrimental effect on the nation.

The situation within Indian states is no different; South Indian states such as Tamil Nadu and Kerala were reported to have a prevalence of 21.9% in 2016, while incidence of prediabetes in Kerala was found to be 36.7% [8]. A prospective study on lifestyle disease from Alleppey, Kerala, found incidence rate of T2DM as 24.5 per 1000 person-years and impaired fasting glucose (IFG) as 45.01 per 1000 persons [9]. The heavy disease burden of diabetes is fuelled by overweight, obesity, inadequate physical activity and unhealthy eating and lifestyle practices. Diabetes is a silent killer which remains asymptomatic at early stages and goes undetected until presented with a vascular event such as angina or myocardial infarction or stroke.

Although insulin is found to be a remedy for diabetes, the place of physical activity is superior to insulin for effective action on insulin receptors. Unfortunately, subjects with diabetes appear to be sedentary or related to disease itself, but exhibit reduced cardiorespiratory fitness [10].

3. Risk factors of Type 2 diabetes

Most of the risk factors except genetic causes are lifestyle-related and thus modifiable. Economic evolution and increased standard of living have replaced bicycle riders and pedestrians with motorized vehicles for quicker transport. Children are discouraged from walking and cycling to school, and commutation is replaced with school bus. Games or physical training sessions are restricted or non-existent in many schools with some schools having no playgrounds at all. Additional tuition classes for high academic achievements and the competition to get admission to schools and colleges take away the after-school play time from children.

Advanced technology and digitalization have changed activity pattern at work and during leisure time to energy-saving measures. Considerable time is spent on sedentary pursuits, with television, movie watching, video games, internet surfing and telephone gossip sessions. The advent of the smartphone has again further contributed to people developing sedentary habits. With the advent of COVID-19 pandemic, smart phone has become an inevitable tool for teaching and learning, exposing the young generation to a prolonged screen time. Pandemic also promoted social isolation, lock down, virtual communication and increased sedentarism. All these have indirectly contributed to physical inactivity and impaired cardiorespiratory fitness.

Significant association was reported with overweight and obesity, while lack of physical activities, prolonged TV watching/playing computer games, frequent consumption of fast food/junk food and frequent consumption of calorie dense food items were found to be contributory factors to developing DM. Higher socioeconomic family status and familial obesity also play a significant role among risk factors [11]. Mendenhall et al. found that the higher-income group conveyed 'tension' or stress associated with children's futures, financial security and family dynamics, whereas depression was most common among the poorest, the middle (38%) and the high-income (29%) group [12]. Significant risk factors for T2DM among adolescents are found to be obesity, positive family history, female gender, puberty and being a low-birth-weight baby. Presence of T2DM among a first- or second-degree relative is reported in 75–100% of patients.

Prevalence of T2DM increased from 36% to 54% when there was a positive family history of diabetes on the non-diabetic parental side also. When both parents were diabetic, the prevalence rate was as high as 62% [13]. Genetics plays a significant role for T2DM in children. Children born to mothers with T2DM are particularly at increased risk for the disease when compared with children whose fathers had T2DM. The risk is higher for boys than for girls. A strong positive family history of diabetes (FHD) is present in 45%–80% of children with T2DM. However, research explains only 10% of the heritability of type 2 DM. The appearance of T2DM at a very young age like childhood and adolescence is distressing as it consumes the most productive years of life, and its consequences on society, public and mental health are dreadful. For a healthy nation and economy, healthy individuals and healthy families are essential.

Socio-economic and cultural factors play an important role in childhood nutrition. Parental ignorance and dependency on various media such as television, radio and print advertising for information also can lead to erroneous food and lifestyle practices.

Fewer working parents have the time and energy to prepare a full meal after working hours. And children of many working parents may be in the care of people who may not be much concerned about their charges due to various reasons. Food is the centre of most celebrations and a reward for desired behaviour. Many families believe that a fat baby is a healthy baby [13]. Not to mention that across the world, with income inequality and cultural norms, food distribution itself across societal strata as well as genders depends on purchasing power too.

Healthy organic food is a hard thing to find even for the affluent in many societies today.

Another scenario is where in urban nuclear families where both parents are working full time or in single-parent homes, children are kept engaged with electronic gadgets or digital games. Several hours may be spent on viewing television and snacking till parents return from work. Fewer children walk to school or play outside to save time and energy or due to safety reasons. In urban residential areas with multistorey buildings, people tend to use a lift. Progressive decline in physical activity is a key feature. Climbing few stairs makes an overweight or obese person short of breath, which is a true reflection of impaired cardiorespiratory fitness.

4. Pathophysiology of DM

Diabetes mellitus is a heterogeneous disorder defined by the presence of hyperglycaemia. Diagnostic criteria for diabetes include the following: (1) a fasting plasma glucose (FPG) of ≥126 mg/dL (7.0 mmol/L); (2) classic symptoms of hyperglycaemia plus a random plasma glucose of ≥200 mg/dL (11.1 mmol/L); (3) a 2-hour plasma glucose level ≥200 mg/dL following a standard 75 g oral glucose load (oral glucose tolerance test [OGTT]); or (4) a glycated haemoglobin (HbA1C) >6.5%. HbA1C(A1C) values reflect average blood glucose levels during the previous 2–3 months.

Hyperglycaemia results from inadequate insulin production or insulin resistance. An increase in the counter-regulatory hormones that oppose the effects of insulin also can result in hyperglycaemia. Type 1 DM is often seen in the younger age group below 30 years with peak incidence at puberty. It is characterized by the autoimmune destruction of pancreatic β cells leading to severe or absolute insulin deficiency, requiring insulin treatment lifelong. Patients present with symptoms of polyuria, polydipsia and weight loss with markedly elevated serum glucose concentrations. Absence of insulin leads to formation of **Ketone bodies** resulting in life-threatening acidosis (diabetic ketoacidosis [**DKA**]) which needs urgent intensive intervention.

Type 2 DM accounts for majority cases of diabetes (90–95%). It has a stronger genetic component; prevalence increases with age, occurring mostly in adults (18% of individuals older than 65 years worldwide and 33% in the United States). **Insulin resistance** is the hallmark of type 2 DM and is frequently (85%) associated with obesity. Increased prevalence of T2DM is associated with increase in obesity, increased insulin resistance as well as a decrease in insulin secretion by the pancreas. These patients are often asymptomatic and not diagnosed until 5–7 years after the actual onset of disease owing to the presence of varying amounts of residual insulin secretion, which prevents severe hyperglycaemia or ketosis. Once diagnosed with type 2 DM, majority (70%) are managed with lifestyle modifications (diet, exercise, weight management) alone or in combination.

After **progressive decline in β-cell function,** the disease manifests as an impairment in the acute insulin release that precedes sustained insulin secretion in response to a meal. Once the β-cell mass declines by 40%–60% owing to **β-cell apoptosis**, patients present with impaired fasting glucose and frank Type 2 DM, respectively. Chronic exposure to elevated free fatty acids, hyperglycaemia (**glucolipotoxicity**) and inflammatory cytokines contribute to impaired β-cell insulin secretion in a background of insulin resistance [14].

On a cellular level, mitochondrial dysfunction occurs which may be due to decreased activity, abnormal size or decreased biogenesis. However, these organelles are highly responsive to the stimulus created by muscle contraction and exercise and have a direct link to insulin action/inaction [15]. In a study among 18 diabetic patients, in vivo mitochondrial function among content and glucose disposal were restored following 12 weeks of exercise training (with 13% increased VO2max) [16].

Obesity is a major driver of the increased prevalence of diabetes and plays a critical role in its pathogenesis. Majority (85%) of patients with type 2 DM are obese. Even a 5–10% weight loss in obese individuals with type 2 DM can ameliorate or even terminate the disorder. Excess nutritional intake from any source eventually leads to increased free fatty acid (FFA) storage as triglyceride in adipose tissue. Subcutaneous tissue is the body's major site of fat storage, but it is unable to expand and accommodate excess lipid in obesity. This leads to increased fat deposit in **visceral (central) adipose tissue,** which promotes insulin resistance owing to its high lipid turnover. **Excess lipolysis** from visceral stores directly feeds FFAs into the liver, thus contributing to hepatic lipid accumulation(**steatosis**), insulin resistance and increased hepatic gluconeogenesis, which raises the level of fasting glucose. Metformin, a first-line therapy for type 2 DM, is particularly effective in reversing these hepatic effects of insulin resistance.

The decreased rate of mitochondrial fat oxidation, excess lipid stores and insulin resistance with advanced ageing results in increased prevalence of type 2 DM. Besides, release of certain factors such as **adiponectin, leptin and inflammatory cytokines** such as **tumour necrosis factor** from visceral adipose in addition to FFA also drives insulin resistance. Hyperinsulinaemia can itself contribute to insulin resistance by downregulating insulin receptor levels and desensitizing downstream pathways.

5. Pathology and pathogenesis of DM

Regardless of origin, all types of diabetes result from a relative deficiency of insulin action. The degree of loss of insulin action determines the resultant metabolic derangements. Since the adipose tissue is highly sensitive to insulin action, low insulin levels suppress the excessive lipolysis and thereby enhance storage of fat. Liver liberates glucose in to circulation as a result of glucagon effects. In order to control the same, higher insulin levels are required. In a non-diabetic, healthy individual, basal levels of insulin activity mediate both these responses.

In a healthy person, the hepatic tissue is superbly responsive to changes in pancreatic insulin secretion owing to its high sensitivity and exposure to elevated levels of insulin in the portal circulation. However, stimulated secretion of additional insulin from the pancreas is required for the skeletal muscle to respond to a glucose load with insulin-mediated glucose uptake. Inability of the skeletal muscle to clear up its share of 85% of glucose due to mild insulin deficiency is reflected by postprandial hyperglycaemia.

When an additional loss of insulin action occurs, glucagon's effects on the liver are insufficiently counter-balanced. In such situation, patients will present with both postprandial hyperglycaemia and fasting hyperglycaemia. Insulin deficiency causes hypertriglyceridemia in diabetes, owing to the increase in VLDL production and a decrease in VLDL clearance as a result of decrease in lipoprotein lipase, the enzyme mediating fatty acid storage in adipose tissue.

Insulin is responsible for amino acid uptake and protein synthesis in muscle. Hence, a decrease in insulin action results in decreased muscle protein synthesis among diabetic patients. Marked insulinopenia such as in type 1 DM can cause a negative nitrogen balance and marked **protein wasting.** Superimposition of stress-induced counter-regulatory hormones on already an insulinopenic state exacerbates the metabolic manifestations of deficient insulin action in both Type 1 and 2 DM. The stress of infection and decrease in insulin action in diabetes result in decreased muscle protein synthesis induced DKA in type 1 DM. In addition to all of the metabolic derangements listed, diabetes causes other chronic, progressive complications that are responsible for the high morbidity and mortality rates associated with this disease.

6. Diabetic complications and its mechanisms

Uncontrolled diabetes damages the nerves and blood vessels causing major organ damage, reduced quality of life, disability, premature morbidity and mortality. It also leads to increased disease burden for the family, community and the nation at large.

6.1 Acute complications

6.1.1 Hyperglycaemia

When elevated glucose levels exceed the renal threshold for glucose reabsorption (approximately 200 mg/dL), **glucosuria** results. This causes an osmotic diuresis manifested clinically by **polyuria**, including **nocturia** resulting in dehydration and subsequent thirst that results in **polydipsia**. Glucosuria can lead to significant loss of calories from urinary glucose losses that can exceed 75 g/day. Polyphagia is followed by uncontrolled hyperglycaemia, the result of excessive caloric consumption. Cardinal symptoms of diabetes are three 'polys': polyuria (excessive urination), polydipsia (excessive thirst) and polyphagia (excessive hunger). These are present in type I DM and symptomatic type II DM patients. Loss of fluid and calories through urine (polyuria) results in weight loss. Changes in the water content of the lens of the eye in response to changes in osmolality can cause blurred vision. In women, glucosuria can lead to an increased incidence of candidal vulvovaginitis. In uncircumcised men, candidal balanitis (a similar infection of the glans penis) can occur.

6.1.2 Diabetic Ketoacidosis (DKA)

DKA can also occur in individuals with type 2 DM, particularly during infections, severe trauma or other causes of stress that increase levels of counter-regulatory hormones, thus producing a state of profound inhibition of insulin action. In the absence of insulin, lipolysis is stimulated, providing fatty acids that are favourably converted to ketone bodies in the liver by unopposed glucagon action. When the compensatory mechanism of osmotic diuresis fails, blood sugar can escalate to average of 500 mg/dL, a state of severe hyperglycaemia. Hyperglycaemia leads to increased osmolality, and an intracellular to extracellular fluid shift, inspired by thirst in an effort to maintain intravascular volume. If the polyuria is not controlled, compensatory mechanism fails to maintain circulating fluid volume. Besides, ketoacidosis is often accompanied by nausea and vomiting, resulting in fluid loss and consecutive dehydration and subsequent reduction in renal blood flow. This leads to reduced ability of the kidneys to excrete glucose. Hypovolemia stimulates counter-regulatory hormones, and it turns out into a vicious cycle. Profound cellular dehydration occurs in response to the marked increase in plasma osmolality. A severe loss of intracellular fluid in the brain leads to coma.

The increase in **ketogenesis** caused by a severe lack of insulin action results in increased serum levels of ketones and ketonuria. During ketoacidosis, liver produces ketone bodies mainly Acetoacetate and **β-hydroxybutyrate**, which are organic acids that cause metabolic acidosis resulting in a decrease in blood pH and serum bicarbonate levels. Partial compensatory mechanisms may increase the respiratory rates to compensate for the metabolic acidosis by reducing PCO2. As a result, when pH level is lower than 7.20, characteristic deep, rapid respirations occur (Kussmaul breathing). Although acetone is a minor product of ketogenesis, the ketosis of DKA is much more severe than ketosis due to starvation. Na^+ is lost in addition to water during the osmotic diuresis accompanying DKA, resulting in low serum sodium. Total body stores of K^+ are also depleted by diuresis and vomiting. Without treatment, K^+ can fall to dangerously low levels, leading to potentially lethal cardiac arrhythmias. Marked hypertriglyceridemia can also accompany DKA because of the increased production and decreased clearance of VLDL that occurs in insulin-deficient states. Nausea and vomiting often accompany DKA, contributing to further dehydration. Abdominal pain, present in 30% of patients, may be due to gastric stasis and distention. DKA is treated by replacing water and electrolytes (Na^+ and K^+) and administering insulin.

6.1.3 Hyperosmolar coma

Decreased fluid intake, an intercurrent illness or elderly, debilitated patients who lack sufficient access to water and have abnormal renal function, thus hindering the clearance of excessive glucose loads and can lead to severe hyperosmolar states in the absence of ketosis in type 2 DM. Profound hyperglycaemia and dehydration occur when presented late; glucose levels often range from 800 to 2400 mg/dL, resulting in a higher incidence of coma. Mortality is 10 times higher than in DKA, which is often precipitated by co-morbidity.

6.1.4 Hypoglycaemia

A dangerous factor limiting the achievement of tight glucose control is a complication of insulin treatment in DM. It can also occur with oral hypoglycaemic drugs that stimulate glucose-independent insulin secretion (e.g. sulfonylureas). Hypoglycaemia often occurs during exercise or with fasting. It can be **neurogenic symptoms,** secondary to central nervous system (CNS)-mediated sympathoadrenal discharge; **adrenergic** (shaking, palpitations, anxiety) and **cholinergic** (sweating, hunger) responses that encourage carbohydrate-seeking behaviour. As glucose drops further, **neuroglycopenic symptoms** may occur from the direct effects of hypoglycaemia on CNS function (confusion, coma). A characteristic set of symptoms (night sweats, nightmares, morning headaches) also accompanies hypoglycaemic episodes that occur during sleep (**nocturnal hypoglycaemia**. Acute treatment of hypoglycaemia in diabetic individuals consists of the rapid oral administration of glucose at the onset of warning symptoms or the intramuscular administration of exogenous glucagon by another person when neuroglycopenic symptoms prohibit oral glucose self-treatment. Excessive glucose administration can lead to rebound hyperglycaemia by the action of counter-regulatory hormones (**Somogyi phenomenon).**

6.2 Chronic complications

Over time, diabetes results in damage and dysfunction in multiple organ systems by damaging the blood vessels and nerves. Both **microvascular disease** (retinopathy, nephropathy, neuropathy) and **macrovascular disease** (coronary artery disease, peripheral vascular disease), which occurs with increased frequency in diabetes, contribute to the high morbidity and mortality rates associated with diabetes mellitus. Peripheral Neuropathy where the sensory perception is impaired due to nerve damage, there is an increased risk of foot ulcers that lead to increased morbidity. Good glycaemic control plays a key role in preventing complications. Genetic factors also clearly play a role in complications.

6.2.1 Microvascular complications

Hyperglycaemia plays a critical role in microvascular disease. The high intracellular levels of glucose in cells that cannot downregulate glucose entry (the endothelium, glomeruli and nerve cells) result in microvascular damage. There is overproduction of mitochondrial-derived reactive oxygen species generated by an increased flux of glucose through the tricarboxylic acid (TCA) cycle. These changes in the microvasculature result in an increase in protein accumulation in vessel walls, endothelial cell dysfunction, loss of endothelial cells and, ultimately, occlusion. The formation of irreversibly glycated proteins called **advanced glycosylation end-products (AGEs)** also causes microvascular damage in diabetes. Elevated glucose leads to increased glycation of HbA within red blood cells. The measurement of HbA1c in diabetic patients serves as an index of glycaemic control over the preceding 3 months.

6.2.2 Retinopathy

Diabetes is a leading cause of blindness in developed countries occurring in two distinct stages: non-proliferative and proliferative. **Microaneurysms** of the retinal capillaries, appearing as tiny red dots, are the earliest clinically detectable sign of diabetic retinopathy (**background retinopathy**). The appearance of hard exudates in the area of the macula is often associated with **macular oedema**, which can occur at any stage of retinopathy progression and is the most common cause of blindness in type 2 DM, occurring in 7% of diabetics. Occlusion of capillaries and terminal arterioles causes areas of retinal ischemia that appear as hazy yellow areas with indistinct borders (**cotton wool spots** or **soft exudates**) at areas of infarction. Retinal haemorrhage can also occur, and retinal veins develop segmental dilation. Retinopathy can progress to a second, more severe stage characterized by the proliferation of new vessels (**proliferative retinopathy).** These capillary vessels are abnormal, and traction between new fibrovascular networks and the vitreous can result in **vitreous haemorrhage** or **retinal detachment**, both are potential causes of blindness in diabetic patients.

6.2.3 Nephropathy

Globally, the most common cause of ESRD is chronic, uncontrolled diabetes. A disordered glomerular function leads to diabetic nephropathy.

Basement membranes of the glomerular capillaries get thickened and obliterate the vessels. The mesangium surrounding the glomerular vessels is increased owing to the deposition of basement membrane-like material and can encroach on the glomerular vessels. The afferent and efferent glomerular arteries become sclerosed. Histological alterations of renal glomeruli are accompanied by early **microalbuminuria**, which is not revealed on a routine urinalysis dipstick method. Albuminuria is thought to be due to a decrease in the heparan sulfate content of the thickened glomerular capillary basement membrane. As the glomerular lesion progresses, proteinuria rises and nephropathy becomes evident. Presence of heavy proteinuria (>300 mg/day) that can be spotted on a routine urine examination signifies diabetic nephropathy. Proteinuria continues to increase as renal function deteriorates. Therefore, ESRD is preceded by massive, nephrotic-range proteinuria (>4 g/d). The presence of hypertension speeds up this process. Hypertension worsens as renal function deteriorates. Therefore, controlling hypertension is critical in preventing the progression of diabetic nephropathy.

6.2.4 Neuropathy

Occurs in about 60% of both type 1 and type 2 DM patients and is a major cause of morbidity. Diabetic neuropathy can be divided into three major types: (a) a distal, primarily sensory, symmetric polyneuropathy the most common (50% incidence); (b) an autonomic neuropathy, occurring frequently in individuals with distal polyneuropathy (>20% incidence); and (c) much less common, transient asymmetric neuropathies involving specific nerves, nerve roots or plexuses.

a. **Symmetric distal polyneuropathy** – The demyelination of peripheral nerves, a hallmark of diabetic polyneuropathy, affects distal nerves preferentially and is usually manifested clinically by a symmetric sensory loss in the distal lower extremities (**stocking distribution**) that is preceded by numbness, tingling and paraesthesias. These symptoms, which begin distally and move proximally, can also occur in the hands (**glove distribution**). Pathologic features of affected peripheral somatic nerves include the demyelination and loss of nerve fibres with reduced axonal regeneration, accompanied by microvascular lesions, including the thickening of basement membranes. In addition, the microvascular disease that accompanies these neural lesions may also contribute to nerve damage.

b. **Mononeuropathy:** Vascular occlusion and ischemia are thought to play a central role in the pathogenesis of these asymmetric focal neuropathies, which are usually of limited duration and occur more frequently in type 2 DM. It is characterized by the abrupt, usually painful onset of motor loss in isolated cranial or peripheral nerves (**mononeuropathy**) or in multiple isolated nerves.

6.3 Macrovascular complications

Accounting for significant morbidity and mortality in both types of diabetes, the effects of large-vessel disease are particularly devastating in type 2 DM and are responsible for approximately 75% of deaths.

6.3.1 Atherosclerosis

Atherosclerotic macrovascular disease commonly occurs in diabetes, resulting in an increased incidence of myocardial infarction, stroke and claudication and gangrene of the lower extremities. The reasons for the increased risk of **atherosclerosis** in diabetes are threefold: (1) traditional risk factors, hypertension and hyperlipidaemia, (2) diabetes itself is an independent risk factor for atherosclerosis; and (3) diabetes when synergized with other known risk factors increases atherosclerosis. Hence, the elimination of other risk factors, therefore, can greatly reduce the risk of atherosclerosis in diabetes.

6.3.2 Hypertension

Hypertension is associated with increased total body extracellular Na+ content and volume expansion which occurs in type 1 DM and type 2 DM. Insulin resistance is associated with activation of the renin-angiotensin system, which leads to hypertension, while renin-angiotensin system activation, in turn, decreases insulin sensitivity. Insulin resistance is central to the pathogenesis of two obesity-associated syndromes: (1) **prediabetes** (e.g., FPG 100–125 mg/dL, A1C 5.7–6.4%); and (2) **metabolic syndrome** (a cluster of metabolic abnormalities, including central obesity [waist ≥102 cm for males or≥88 cm for females], elevated glucose [≥100 mg/dL], elevated blood pressure [≥130/≥85 mm Hg], elevated triglycerides [≥150 mg/dL] and low high-density lipoprotein [HDL] cholesterol [<40 mg/dL]). Both syndromes are associated with increased cardiovascular risk, as well as an increased risk for the later development of diabetes. The **Diabetes Prevention Programme** has demonstrated that significant risk reductions for the development of type 2 DM occur in response to lifestyle interventions in this population.[1] **Hypertriglyceridemia**, which is associated with an increased risk of cardiovascular disease. The compositions of LDL and HDL are altered by elevated levels of VLDL. It also transfers triglycerides to these particles, depletes them of cholesterol and creates **small, dense LDL particles** and **low HDL** cholesterol levels. Eventually, both of these are independent risk factors for cardiovascular disease. Treatment of hyperglycaemia does not normalize lipid profiles in obese, insulin-resistant individuals with type 2 DM unless accompanied by weight reduction treatment.

6.3.3 Diabetic foot ulcers

Symmetric polyneuropathy (present in 75–90% of diabetics with foot ulcers) results in insensate feet among diabetics, which makes them highly susceptible to foot injuries. Once developed, it is less amenable to regular healing, and the wound may get complicated by osteomyelitis and result in amputation in 1%, an event associated with high mortality (50% by 3 years). Other reasons for diabetic foot ulcers are macrovascular disease (present in 30–40% of those with foot ulcers) and microvascular disease; infections caused by alterations in neutrophil function and vascular

---

[1] Diabetes Prevention Program Research Group. Long-term effects of lifestyle intervention or metformin on diabetes development and microvascular complications over 15-year follow-up: the Diabetes Prevention Program Outcomes Study Diabetes Prevention Program Research Group† Show footnotes. The Lancet Diabetes and Endocrinology [Internet]. VOLUME 3, ISSUE 11, P866-875, NOVEMBER 01, 2015. Available from: https://www.thelancet. com/journals/landia/article/PIIS2213-8587(15)00291-0/fulltext

insufficiency; and faulty wound healing. Unfortunately, about 10% of diabetics develop diabetic foot ulcers.

6.3.4 Infection

Abnormal cell-mediated immunity, defective neutrophil chemotaxis and phagocytosis, reduced blood flow from vascular lesions prevent inflammatory cells reaching wound sites, making them prone to infections which often become severe infection. Candidal infections, periodontal disease, necrotizing papillitis, mucormycosis and malignant otitis externa caused by Pseudomonas aeruginosa are common infections that occur in diabetics.

Skeletal changes in diabetes – Adults with type 2 DM have a 40–70% increased fracture risk, perhaps owing to increased cortical porosity. Bone fragility in diabetes is considered as an additional factor attributable to microvascular disease [17].

7. Measures to maintain Cardiorespiratory fitness (CRF)

Enhanced Physical Activity (PA) was and continues to be a cornerstone of diabetes prevention and management. Regular aerobic exercise at modest levels (<6METs) can lessen HbA1c by almost 0.7% and improve insulin sensitivity while keeping weight unchanged [18]. In other words, 1-week aerobic exercise can improve your body's sensitivity to insulin in peripheral tissues irrespective of insulin usage. Optimally, subjects with diabetes should engage in regular PA on a daily basis, and the shorter the exposure to PA, the higher the effort is needed to get the same effect on insulin sensitivity for lasting effect [19].

Physical activity or exercise can be classified broadly as aerobic or anaerobic. Physical activity refers to energy expenditure above resting stage while exercises is a type of planned, structured and repetitive bodily activity aimed at improving physical fitness. Physical activity or exercise can be classified broadly as aerobic or anaerobic. Aerobic activity refers to repetitive, low-intensity, long-duration movements that apply large muscle groups utilizing aerobic energy pathways using fatty acids as substrate. Specifically, chronic exposure to aerobic exercises of adequate intensity and duration leads to increased aerobic capacity or cardiorespiratory fitness (CRF). CRF is typically reported as metabolic equivalents (METs), with one MET defined as the amount of oxygen consumption at rest (3.5 ml O2/kg/min).

Today's lifestyle marked by prosperous socioeconomic status, sedentariness and obesity have made significant contributions as independent risk factors for T2DM. Encouraging reasonable dynamic physical activity for 150 min/week can typically reduce health risks associated with numerous chronic illnesses and their prevention.

Irrespective of sedentary lifestyle and duration of the disease, individuals with diabetes exhibit exercise intolerance with subnormal cardiorespiratory fitness, owing to certain vascular abnormalities and slowed kinetics for oxygen uptake.

Older adults with DM2 have greater muscle mass loss, reduced upper and lower body strength, increased visceral adiposity and increased disability [20–22]. Poorly controlled DM2 patients have, in addition, poor capillary recruitment during skeletal contraction [23]. Resistance Training (RT) has largest effect on the musculoskeletal measurements such as muscle strength [24], can significantly improve insulin sensitivity, glycaemic control including HbA1c, increase fat-free mass, reduce the requirement for diabetes medications, reduce abdominal adiposity and improve cardiovascular risk markers [25–27].

Resistance exercise training (RT) is a promising strategy to promote overall metabolic health in individuals with T2DM, with improvements in muscle mitochondrial performance, increase in muscle mass, positive impact insulin responsiveness and glucose control [28]. Current guidelines for DM2 prevention and management recommend at least 150 min per week of MVPA and an additional two (ideally three) resistance sessions per week (at least 60 min). Besides, breaking up of prolonged sedentary time with light walking promises with improved glycaemic parameters. The duration of DM2 is associated with response to exercise. Resistance training may benefit patients with long-standing DM2, having more extreme exercise intolerance, muscle weakness and sarcopenia.

8. Conclusion

Poor Cardiorespiratory Fitness (CRF) is a well-established independent predictor of Cardiovascular Disease and overall mortality among subjects with prediabetes, DM1 and DM2. Increased Physical Activity (PA) and higher CRF offer metabolic health benefits for DM2 patients in proportion to the level of fitness independent of BMI. Increases in Physical Activity patterns have emerged as an integral part of the prevention and management supported by a multitude of reproducible randomized studies confirming the strong link to enhanced CRF. Significant implementation challenges are, however, the bottom being adherence, therapeutic regimens should be designed to improve CRF in a society where a profound lifestyle shift has taken place dominated by non-exercise PA and sedentary behaviours. Being a modifiable risk factor, a healthcare provider prescription for enhanced fitness is perhaps using CRF as a vital sign. Involvement of progressive societal and political encounter via education and support for alternatives to transportation, creating more appropriate indoor and outdoor architecture harm from emerging exposure risks from pollution is an indispensable component of promoting physical activity for better CRF in the population particularly for those who are at risk of noncommunicable diseases such as DM and hypertension. This will bring significant reduction in excessive economic burden of diabetes and reduce premature mortality and morbidity among existing diabetics and prediabetics. Prevention is better than cure.

9. A word of caution: preventive measures to save the budding generation

India, being a developing country, has over 253 million adolescents who need to be protected from premature morbidity and mortality through health education and creating a favourable environment to adopt an active healthy lifestyle. They should be motivated to exercise, avoid high calorie food habits and maintain a healthy BMI. Government should develop policies to allow provision for healthy meals and snacks in hotels and restaurants, cancellation of license for junk food sale at all types of food outlets, providing warning signs about unhealthy food consumption, etc. Also, promotion policies such as reduced insurance premium for people with normal BMI, healthy food habits and regular health check-ups. Provision for exercise and healthy food habits should be provided mandatorily at all working places in order to facilitate 150 minutes of physical exercise a week. The same should be mandatorily implemented at all schools and colleges. The recognition and licences should be tagged with these requirements to create public awareness on the importance of controlling and preventing diabetes mellitus.

Ensure availability of healthy groceries, vegetables and fruits at markets, healthy food items at shopping malls and restaurants, canteens and hostels to promote healthy eating habits among the public. At present, all restaurants and bakeries as well as small food outlets provide high-calorie sweetened and oily foods, highly processed foods that are attractive to the population, particularly the youngsters. Strong awareness about dangers of obesity and NCDs such as DM, HT and cancer along with provision for healthy meal will encourage more than 50% of population to adopt healthy eating habits.

"An ounce of prevention is worth a pound of cure!"
Benjamin Franklin

Conflict of interest

Nil.

Author details

Theyamma Joseph[1,2]* and Jacquline C. Vadasseril[3]

1 JJT University, Rajasthan, India

2 Mar Sleeva College of Nursing, Kottayam, Kerala, India

3 Bishop Vayalil Medical Centre, Moolamattom, Kerala, India

*Address all correspondence to: princimbcn@gmail.com

References

[1] WHO Health Statistics. 2021. Available from: https://www. nwho. int/ health topics/ diabetes#tab=tab1

[2] Kokkinos P, Narayan P. Cardiorespiratory fitness in Cardiometabolic diseases, Prevention and Management in Clinical Practice. 1st ed. Washington DC: Springer; 2022. pp. 80-82

[3] van Dieren S, Beulens JW, van der Schouw YT, Grobbee DE, Neal B. The global burden of diabetes and its complications: An emerging pandemic. European Journal of Cardiovascular Preventive Rehabilitation. 2010;**17** (Suppl. 1):S3-S8

[4] American Diabetes Association. Cardiovascular disease and risk management. Diabetes Care. 2017;**40**:S75-S87

[5] Tao Z, Shi A, Zhao J. Epidemiological perspectives of diabetes. Cell Biochemistry and Biophysics. 2015;**73**:1

[6] Pradeepa R. Epidemiology of type 2 diabetes in India. Indian Journal of Ophthalmology. 2020;**69**:2932-2938

[7] Mandaviya M. Union Minister of Health and Family Welfare to the Lok Sabha on December 3. 2021

[8] Nanditha A, Snehalatha C, Satheesh K, Susairaj P, Simon M, Vijaya L, et al. Secular TRends in DiabEtes in India (STRiDE-I): Change in prevalence in 10 years among urban and rural populations in Tamil Nadu. Diabetes Care. 2019;**42**:476-485

[9] Vijayakumar G, Manghat S, Vijayakumar R, Simon L, Scaria LM, Vijayakumar A, et al. Incidence of type 2 diabetes mellitus and prediabetes in Kerala, India: Results from a 10-year prospective cohort. BMC Public Health. 2019;**19**:140

[10] Henson J, Dunstan DW, Davies MJ, Yates T. Sedentary behaviour as a new behavioural target in the prevention and treatment of type 2 diabetes. Diabetes Metabolic Research Review. 2016;**32**(Suppl. 1):213-220

[11] Mistry SK, Puthussery S. Risk factors of overweight and obesity in childhood and adolescence in South Asian countries: A systematic review of the evidence. Public Health. 2015 Mar;**129**(3):200-209

[12] Mendenhall E, Shivashankar R, Tandon N, Ali MK, Venkat Narayan KM, Prabhakaran D. Stress and diabetes in socioeconomic context: A qualitative study of urban Indians. Social Science & Medicine. Dec 2012;**75**(12):2522-2529

[13] Joseph T. Effectiveness of a Structured Teaching Programme on Knowledge and Lifestyle Practices Related to Prevention of T2DM among Adolescents in Selected Schools of Kerala. Bangalore, Karnataka: Rajiv Gandhi University of Health Sciences; 2017

[14] Funk JL. Disorders of the endocrine pancreas. In: Gary DH, Stephen JM, editors. Pathophysiology of Disease: An Introduction to Clinical Medicine. 8th ed. New York: McGraw-Hill Education; 2019. pp. 1251-1286

[15] Nylén ES, Kokkinos P. Physical activity, cardiorespiratory fitness, and the diabetes spectrum. In: Kokkinos P, Narayan P, editors. Cardiorespiratory Fitness in Cardiometabolic Diseases: Prevention and Management in Clinical

Practice. 1st ed. Switzerland AG: Springer; 2019. pp. 191-206

[16] Meex RCR, Schrauwen-Hinderling VB, Moonen Kornips E, Schaart G, Mensink M, Phielix E, et al. Restoration of muscle mitochondrial function and metabolic flexibility in type 2 diabetes by exercise training is paralleled by increased myocellular fat storage and improved insulin sensitivity. Diabetes. 2010;**59**:572-579

[17] Diabetes Prevention Program Research Group. Long-term effects of lifestyle intervention or metformin on diabetes development and microvascular complications over 15-year follow-up: The Diabetes Prevention Program Outcomes Study Diabetes Prevention Program Research Group† Show footnotes. The Lancet Diabetes and Endocrinology. 2015;**3**:866-875

[18] Winnick JJ, Sherman WM, Habash DL, Stout MB, Failla ML, Belury MA, et al. Short-term aerobic exercise training in obese humans with type 2 diabetes mellitus improves whole-body insulin sensitivity through gains in peripheral, not hepatic insulin sensitivity. Journal of Clinical Endocrinology Metabolism. 2008;**93**:771-778

[19] Yardley JE, Alberga A, Kenny GP, Sigal RJ. Lifestyle issues: Exercise. In: RIG H, Cockram CS, Flyvbjerg A, Goldstein BJ, editors. Textbook of Diabetes. 4th ed. London: Wiley-Blackwell; 2010. pp. 358-379

[20] Vandervoort AA. Aging of the human neuromuscular system. Muscle Nerve. 2002;**25**:17-25

[21] Park SW, Goodpaster BH, Strotmeyer ES, et al. Decreased muscle strength and quality in older adults with type 2 diabetes: The health, aging, and body composition study. Diabetes. 2006;**55**:1813-1818

[22] Seok WP, Goodpaster BH, Jung SL, et al. Excessive loss of skeletal muscle mass in older adults with type 2 diabetes. Diabetes Care. 2009;**32**:1993-1997

[23] Womack L, Peters D, Barrett EJ, Kaul S, Price W, Lindner JR. Abnormal skeletal muscle capillary recruitment during exercise in patients with type 2 diabetes mellitus and microvascular complications. Journal of American College of Cardiology. 2009;**53**:2175-2183

[24] Hovanec N, Sawant A, Overend TJ, Petrella RJ, Vandervoort AA. Resistance training and older adults with type 2 diabetes mellitus: Strength of the evidence. Journal of Aging Research. 2012;**2012**:284635

[25] Castaneda C, Layne JE, Munoz-Orians L, Gordon PL, Walsmith J, Foldvari M, et al. A randomized controlled trial of resistance exercise training to improve glycaemic control in older adults with type 2 diabetes. Diabetes Care. 2002;**25**:2335-2341

[26] Brooks N, Layne JE, Gordon PL, Roubenoff R, Nelson ME, Castaneda-Sceppa C. Strength training improves muscle quality and insulin sensitivity in Hispanic older adults with type 2 diabetes. International Journal of Medical Science. 2007;**4**:19-27

[27] Dunstan DW, Daly RM, Owen N. High-intensity resistance training improves glycaemic control in older patients with type 2 diabetes. Diabetes Care. 2002;**25**:1729-1736

[28] Pesta DH, Goncalves RLS, Madiraju AK, Strasser B, Sparks LM. Resistance training to improve type 2 diabetes: Working toward a prescription for the future. Nutritional Metabolism. 2017;**14**:24

Chapter 9

Relation between Vastus Lateralis Electromyography Activation and VO_{2max} Values Obtained in Bicycle Ergometry

Hasan Sözen

Abstract

The study aimed to investigate the relationship between maximum oxygen consumption values obtained on a bicycle ergometer and vastus lateralis (VL) muscle EMG activity values during the test. A total of 20 athletes participated in the study. To determine the VO_{2max}, a bicycle ergometer was used with a portable gas analyzer. The discontinuous incremental protocol was used to determine the VO_{2max} values of subjects. The data were gathered from the right side VL muscle *via* surface electromyography. According to the results obtained, MVIC% values of the VL muscle of the subjects and VO_{2max} (mL min^{-1}) values ($p = 0.586$, $r = 0.130$); VO_{2max} (mL min^{-1} kg^{-1}) values ($p = 0.295$, $r = 0.246$); RER values ($p = 0.308$, $r = -0.240$) and HRmax (beats min^{-1}) values ($p = 0.321$, $r = 0.234$) were not statistically significant and no significant difference was found in the regression analysis between the MVIC% value of the VL muscle obtained and the VO_{2max} (mL min^{-1} kg^{-1}) values ($p = 0.295$, $R^2 = 0.061$). There was no significant correlation and regression between the muscle activation involved in the workout during the VO_{2max} test and the cardiovascular response.

Keywords: VO_{2max}, aerobic capacity, muscle activation, bicycle exercise, electromyography

1. Introduction

To provide the oxygen necessary for the increased metabolic rate during exercise, an increase in respiratory volume frequency occurs. Maximal exercises can also increase to 200 lt/min. This is achieved by increasing the respiratory volume and frequency. On the other hand, while the respiratory minute volume can reach 200 lt/min in trained athletes during exercises performed with the same intensity, it is 100 lt/min in inactive individuals (sedentary). This is related to the fact that training strengthens the respiratory muscles in trained individuals. There is no significant change in respiratory volume and frequency with training. However, with training, there is an increase in the oxygen consumption rate (VO_{2max}) in the maximal aerobic metabolism in the tissues. Whether the person is trained or not, if there is no disease, he can always get much more oxygen than the body needs. Therefore, the important factor is to increase the availability of oxygen through training, in other words, to increase the VO_{2max} level in the tissues.

The most obvious effect of training on athletes is to increase oxygen diffusion capacity. Oxygen diffusion capacity is an indicator of the diffusion rate of oxygen from the alveoli to the blood. With regular training, respiratory volume in athletes does not change much in rest and submaximal exercises, but a significant increase is observed in maximal exercise. This significant increase is also seen in respiratory frequency and respiratory minute volume.

Acute physiological responses to changes in exercise intensity provide comprehensive information about the functional capacity and exercise tolerance of healthy individuals and patient populations. The integration of central and peripheral physiological systems determines the relationship between oxygen demand and allows the individual to adapt to changes in metabolic demand [1]. Among the physiological parameters, the maximum oxygen consumption is an indicator that gives information about the level of cardiovascular fitness and the functionality of the cardiovascular system [2]. The maximal oxygen volume level used by the skeletal muscles during a progressively increased exercise test is defined as maximum oxygen volume. VO_{2max} is a good indicator of aerobic capacity and is an indicator of the physiological integration of pulmonary, cardiovascular, and neuromuscular functions [3]. Aerobic metabolism during isometric or dynamic activities is estimated by indirect calorimetry, using oxygen and carbon dioxide gas exchange, where the energy used by working muscles reflects changes in pulmonary oxygen uptake [4]. Unfortunately, metabolic power measures based on a gas exchange cannot resolve metabolic costs to a higher resolution than breathing rate. As a result, information about muscle contractions that affect metabolic strength is neglected because these contractions may occur more frequently than breathing rate [5]. The maximum rate of O_2 intake (i.e., VO_{2max}) measured during large muscle mass exercises such as cycling or running is considered the gold standard measure of integrated cardiopulmonary-muscle oxidative function. The development of fast-responding gas analyzers that allow the measurement of breath-by-breath pulmonary gas exchange and progressive maximum exercise tests that increase rapidly or increase continuously with ramp test protocols are often used in clinical and experimental research. The VO_{2max} estimate obtained after these tests is sometimes not sufficient alone [6]. For this reason, many researchers resort to secondary criteria such as respiratory exchange rate, maximal heart rate, and/or maximal blood lactate concentration, which can result in VO_{2max}. However, studies examining the relationship between VO_{2max} values and activations of primary working muscles are limited [7].

Strength changes during muscle contractions are primarily reached by changing the number of active motor units and motor unit ignition rates. These changes can be detected using surface electromyography (EMG), which provides information about the active muscle by measuring the electrical signals of the motor unit action potentials. EMG fluctuates significantly within milliseconds during isotonic movements. Therefore, EMG should contain information about metabolic strength at a higher temporal resolution than gas exchange measures, but it is not known whether EMG can be used to predict (isometric) metabolic power changes during steady-state dynamic activities. However, the most important value that can be obtained from EMG during these isometric activities is muscle fatigue indices [8]. Surface EMG (sEMG) is widely used to measure the magnitude and timing of muscle activation during a variety of physical tasks, which has wide application in sports science research. sEMG's ability to analyze dynamic situations gives it a special interest in sports. Improving the efficiency of a movement involves the proper use of muscles, both in terms of effort savings and effectiveness, as well as injury prevention. In particular, the performance of a task can be improved in terms of muscle activation and/or muscle fatigue based on analysis of the frequency of electromyographic traces observed. It should be noted that although EMG is an indicator of muscular effort in a particular action, it does not provide us with muscle strength parameters. In this regard, it is important to emphasize that the relationship between EMG activity and effort is only qualitative. Recently, experiments have been carried out on applications for purposes such as the evaluation of muscle fiber type and the characterization of muscles in the field of sports [9].

In this context, this study aimed to investigate the EMG activation of the VL muscle, which is the primary muscle involved in the workout with VO_{2max} values a cardiovascular response during cycling exercise.

The hypothesis of the study is that there is a relation between individuals' VO_2 values and actively working muscle EMG values.

2. Material and methods

2.1 Study participants

Twenty active athletes' volunteer subjects (10 females, 10 males) participated in the study (**Table 1**). Volunteers participate in any sportive activity at least 3 days a week and have similar performance levels. The inclusion criteria of the volunteers participating in the study were determined as follows:

- Having dominant legs right,
- Participating in any sporting activity at least 3 days a week,
- Not having any joint injury in the last 6 months,
- Does not interfere with exercising for cycling,
- Not using caffeine-type stimulants on the day of the study,
- Not smoking,
- Being a volunteer.

All participants approved the volunteering form. The study was conducted by the principles of the latest Helsinki Declaration upon receiving the necessary permissions.

2.2 VO_{2max} measurement

To determine the VO_{2max}, a bicycle ergometer (Monark 839E, Monark Ltd., Varberg, Sweden) was used with a portable gas analyzer (K5, Cosmed, Rome, Italy) and heart rate monitor (Cosmed, Rome, Italy). Discontinuous incremental protocol

Variables	Female (n = 10)	Male (n = 10)	Total (n = 20)
Age (years)	19.7 ± 1.15	19.9 ± 0.87	19.8 ± 0.22
Height (cm)	166.6 ± 3.02	174.7 ± 9.33	170.6 ± 1.77
Weight (kg)	56.7 ± 4.69	72.7 ± 7.00	64.7 ± 2.24
BMI (kg/m^2)	20.4 ± 1.6	23.7 ± 1.64	22.0 ± 0.53

Abbreviations: BMI; body mass index.
Values are presented as mean ± SD.

Table 1.
General characteristics of subjects.

(DP) was used to determine the VO_{2max} values of subjects [10]. DP protocol concerned five workloads of 5 min each, interspersed by at least 5 minutes. Basal measurements were recorded with the participants standing on the bicycle ergometer. The first two workloads were set at 50 W and 100 W for all participants. The following three workloads were tailored for each participant according to the individual cardiorespiratory responses to the first two workloads and considering the theoretical maximum heart rate determined. Firstly, based on the VO_2 and the heart rate recorded during the first two stages, a submaximal linear regression was determined up to the predicted peak heart rate, to predict the speed corresponding to possible exhaustion. Then, the third, fourth, and fifth workloads corresponded to approximately 80%, 90%, and 105% of the predicted peak workload, respectively. The fourth and fifth workloads were recalculated using the heart rate and VO_2 recorded during the third and fourth stages, respectively [11]. The last stage was tailored to let the participants maintain the task for at least 4 min.

2.3 EMG measurement

In the study, the vastus lateralis (VL) muscle, which is one of the most active muscles during cycling exercise [12], was studied. EMG measurements of the VL muscles were recorded during the VO_{2max} test. EMG signals of the right leg were recorded. A Noraxon DTS wireless system (Noraxon Telemyo DTS System, Scottsdale, USA) was used for EMG recordings. Dual Ag/AgCl EMG electrodes (spacing—2.0 cm) were placed on the central points of the VL muscle in a parallel fashion to their muscle fibrils according to SENIAM (Surface Electromyography for the Noninvasive Assessment of Muscle) recommendations. Before the electrodes were placed, they were cleaned with an alcohol solution to prevent artifacts, and the skin was shaved to make it smooth [13–15]. After placing the electrodes, the impedance was observed to be within the acceptable range (<50 kOhms).

Raw EMG signals were processed *via* the Noraxon MyoResearch XP Master Edition software (Noraxon, Scottsdale, USA). All EMG signals were filtered using a 500 Hz low-pass filter. The signals were rectified and smoothed using a root mean square (RMS) algorithm (150 ms window).

The maximum value of three Maximal Voluntary Isometric Contraction (MVIC) trials for every 5 s was used for normalization of the EMG data obtained during the exercises. For the $VO2_{max}$ test condition, a peak signal amplitude for VL was determined and divided by the MVIC value for VL. A normalized EMG (nEMG) as MVIC% was used for statistical analysis.

2.4 Statistical analysis

The sample size was reached as a result of power analysis. The data were normally distributed. Obtained VO_{2max} values (VO_{2max} (mL min^{-1}), VO_{2max} (mL min^{-1} kg^{-1}), RER (respiratory exchange ratio), HR_{max} (beats min^{-1}), MVIC%) were tabulated and the arithmetic mean was found and, correlation and regression analysis of all values obtained using SPSS 22 statistics program with MVIC% values of the subjects participating in the test were performed.

3. Results

The values obtained during the VO_{2max} test of the male and female athletes participating in the study and the VL muscle activation values obtained during the test are shown in **Tables 2** and **3**.

Correlation and regression analysis results for the relationship between the values obtained from VO_{2max} measurement of all subjects and EMG muscle activation values obtained from VL muscle are given below.

According to the results obtained, MVIC% values of the VL muscle of the subjects and VO_{2max} (mL min^{-1}) values ($r_{(18)} = 0.130$, $p = 0.586$); VO_{2max} (mL min^{-1} kg^{-1}) values ($r_{(18)} = 0.246$, $p = 0.295$); RER values ($r_{(18)} = -0.240$, $p = 0.308$) and HRmax (beats min^{-1}) values ($r_{(18)} = 0.234$, $p = 0.321$) were not statistically significant in correlation analysis.

According to the result obtained, MVIC% values of the VL muscle of the subjects and VO_{2max} (mL min^{-1}) values ($R^2 = 0.017$, $p = 0.586$); VO_{2max} (mL min^{-1} kg^{-1}) values ($R^2 = 0.061$, $p = 0.295$); RER values ($R^2 = 0.058$, $p = 0.308$); HRmax

Values	N	Min	Max	X	SD
VO_{2max} (mL min^{-1})	10	2371.35	3838.89	3074.59	420.81
VO_{2max} (mL min^{-1} kg)	10	45.60	65.09	54.57	6.93
RER	10	0.98	1.26	1.12	0.08
HR_{max} (beats min^{-1})	10	159.00	187.00	176.34	11.77
MVIC%	10	59.12	132.40	85.76	22.64

Table 2.
Values of female athletes participating in the study.

Values	N	Min	Max	X	SD
VO_{2max} (mL min^{-1})	10	4419.77	5993.39	5348.50	461.35
VO_{2max} (mL min^{-1} kg)	10	67.78	78.33	72.02	3.75
RER	10	1.13	1.26	1.16	0.04
HR_{max} (beats min^{-1})	10	162.00	194.00	184.10	12.40
MVIC%	10	78.71	121.60	93.08	12.09

Table 3.
Values of male athletes participating in the study.

(beats min^{-1}) values ($R^2 = 0.055$, $p = 0.321$) were not statistically significant in the regression analysis.

4. Discussion

In this study, muscle activation of VL and VO_{2max} values were compared during the VO_{2max} test on the bicycle. During cycling exercises, the VL muscle is one of the most involved muscles. VL muscle, which is one of the quadriceps muscles, cannot be neglected, especially during cycling exercise [16]. As a result of the tests and statistical data, no significant correlation was found between VO_{2max} and VL muscle activation values. In the VO_{2max} test performed with the discontinuous incremental protocol, cardiovascular responses and increases in muscle activation were observed at each loading but with this VO_2, muscle activation increased linear rupture. Lactic acid may play a dominant role in a linear rupture in the relationship between muscle activation and VO_2. Exercise-induced intracellular acidosis reduces the capacity of muscle fibers involved in producing work. Acidosis affects muscle activation, with a decrease in pH level. Alternatively, a disruption in myocyte membrane potential due to insufficient Na^+/K^+ pump activity might lead to impairment of excitation-contraction coupling regardless of pH [17]. In a study by Bearden and Moffatt [18], they could not find a linear relationship between VO_2 and power functions. This result is like our study. In a study by Sasaki et al. [19], a significant decrease was observed in the regression slope for VL muscle during cycling exercise, while an increase in the regression slope was observed in the biceps femoris and gastrocnemius muscles. VO_2 is not a linear function of power. During an incremental test, neuromuscular activity and VO_2 increase faster during heavy exercise. Both VO_2 and neuromuscular activity can show a break that can point to an upper limit for sustainable exercise at a very high-power output. Therefore, a similar study can be tried in different VO_{2max} test protocols.

5. Conclusions

According to the results obtained in the study with the hypothesis that there may be a relationship between muscular strain and oxygen consumption, there was no relationship between the oxygen consumption test used to determine the cardiorespiratory endurance of the individual in sports sciences and the EMG test used to determine muscle activation during movement. It can be suggested that future studies should be done on different exercise types and with more subjects.

Conflict of interest

No conflict of interest was declared by the author.

Financial disclosure

The author declared that this study has received no financial support.

Notes/thanks/other declarations

The author thanks all the participants involved in the study, for their patience and committed involvement.

Acronyms and abbreviations

EMG	electromyography
sEMG	surface electromyography
nEMG	normalized electromyography
SENIAM	surface electromyography for the noninvasive assessment of muscle
VL	vastus lateralis
DP	discontinuous incremental protocol
MVIC	maximal voluntary isometric contraction
VO_{2max}	maximal oxygen consumption
RER	respiratory exchange ratio
HR	heart rate

Author details

Hasan Sözen
Ordu University Sport Sciences Faculty, Ordu, Türkiye

*Address all correspondence to: sozenhasan@yahoo.com

References

[1] Boone J, Barstow TJ, Celie B, Prieur F, Bourgois J. The impact of pedal rate on muscle oxygenation, muscle activation, and whole-body VO_2 during ramp exercise in healthy subjects. European Journal of Applied Physiology. 2015;**115**:57-70. DOI: 10.1007/s00421-014-2991-x

[2] Donnelly JE, Blair SN, Jakicic JM, Manore MM, Rankin JW, Smith BK. Appropriate physical activity intervention strategies for weight loss and prevention of weight regain for adults. Medicine & Science Sports & Exercise. 2009;**41**:459-471

[3] Sözen H, Akyıldız C. The effects of aerobic and anaerobic training on aerobic and anaerobic capacity. The Journal of International Anatolia Sport Science. 2018;**3**(3):331-337

[4] Poole DC, Gaesser GA, Hogan MC, Knight DR, Wagner PD. Pulmonary and leg VO2 during submaximal exercise: Implications for muscular efficiency. Journal of Applied Physiology. 1992;**72**(2):805-810

[5] Blake OM, Wakeling JM. Estimating changes in metabolic power from EMG. Springerplus. 2013;**2**:229

[6] Poole DC, Andrew MJ. Measurement of the maximum oxygen uptake VO2max: VO2peak is no longer acceptable. Journal of Applied Physiology. 2017;**122**(4):997-1002

[7] Halder A. Evaluation of Physical Work Capacity and Leg Muscle Fatigue during Exhaustive Stair Ascending Evacuation. Sweden: Lund University; 2017

[8] Sözen H, Erdogan E, Ince A, Soylu AR. Determination of electromyography-based coordinated fatigue levels in agonist and antagonist muscles of the thigh during squat press exercise. Annals of Applied Sport Science. 2019;**7**(3):21-30

[9] Türker H, Sözen H. Surface electromyography in sports and exercise. Electrodiagnosis in New Frontiers of Clinical Research. 2013;**2013**:175-194

[10] Riboli A, Rampichini S, Ce E, Limonta E, Coratella G, Esposito F. Effect of ramp slope on different methods to determine lactate threshold in semi-professional soccer players. Research in Sports Medicine. 2019;**27**(3):326-338

[11] Riboli A, Emiliano C, Rampichini S, Venturelli M, Alberti G, Limonta E, et al. Comparison between continuous and discontinuous incremental treadmill test to assess velocity at VO2max. The Journal of Sports Medicine and Physical Fitness. 2017;**57**(9):1119-1125

[12] Akima H, Kinugasa R, Kuno S. Recruitment of the thigh muscles during sprint cycling by muscle functional magnetic resonance imaging. International Journal of Sports Medicine. 2005;**26**(04):245-252

[13] Konrad P. The ABC of EMG – A Practical Introduction to Kinesiological Electromyography. Arizona, USA: Noraxon; 2005

[14] De Luca CJA. Practicum on the Use of sEMG Signals in Movement Sciences. Tech. Rep. Boston, MA, USA: Delsys Inc.; 2008

[15] Criswell E. CRAM's Introduction to Surface Electromyography. 2nd ed. London, England: Jones and Bartlett Publishers; 2011

[16] Shinohara M, Moritan T. Increase in neuromuscular activity and oxygen

uptake during heavy exercise. The Annals of Physiological Anthropology. 1992;**11**(3):257-262

[17] Clausen T, Nielsen OB, Harrison AP, Flatman JA, Overgaard K. The Na^+, K^+ pump, and muscle excitability. Acta Physiologica Scandinavica. 1998;**162**(3):183-190

[18] Bearden SE, Moffatt RJ. Leg electromyography and the VO~ 2-power relationship during bicycle ergometry. Medicine and Science in Sports and Exercise. 2001;**33**(7):1241-1245

[19] Sasaki K, Kimura T, Kojima S, Higuchi H. The temporal relationship of thresholds between muscle activity and ventilation during bicycle ramp exercise in community-dwelling elderly males. Journal of Physical Therapy Science. 2016;**28**(11):3213-3219